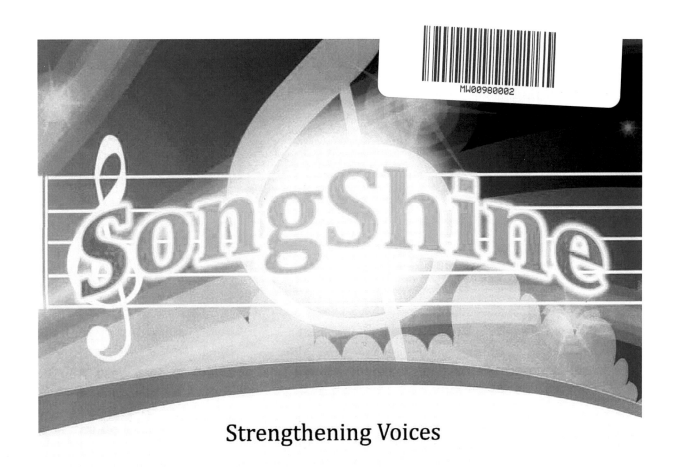

Strengthening Voices

Lifting Spirits

Touching Hearts

Releasing Memories

Creating Community

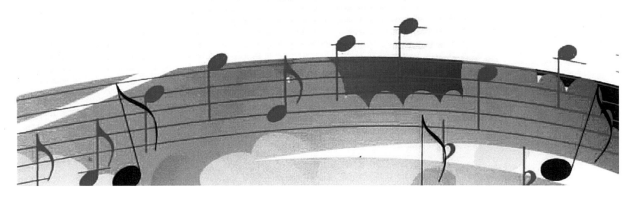

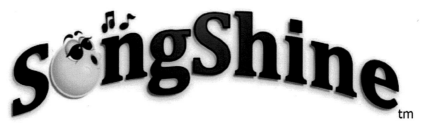

Gaining Vocal Strength Through the Power of Music!

A vocal therapy course for neurological disorders and aging voices.

Copyright © 2010 By Ruthanna Metzgar
www.summitsinger@earthlink.net
All Rights Reserved

Library of Congress
Certificate of Registration # SR 666-664

Published by

Ruthanna Metzger

Printed By

Bayshore Office Products, Inc.

603 Commercial Ave.
Anacortes, Washington 98221
800-221-2124
360-293-4669
www.bayshoreoffice.com

Printing History
November 2010
February 2011

Cover Design: Jeanne Torres

Printed in the United States of America

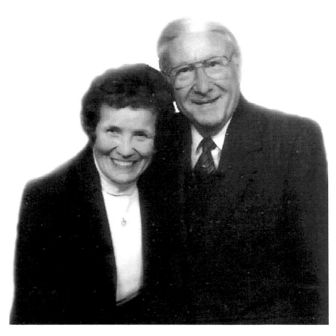

Dedication

A deep debt of gratitude and sincere thanks belong to my parents. My mother, Mildred Ruth Alexander, was a career librarian. She shared with me her love of books and brought home the extra income that paid for my music lessons. My father, Henry Clay Alexander, a pastor, had a passion for people, zest for life, and a love of music. His lively piano playing and joyous singing kept our home ringing, and even during his long journey into Alzheimer's, he never lost his ability to laugh, pray and sing. To their memory I dedicate this work.

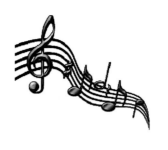

My Own Thoughts

What are my goals in taking SongShine?

_____

_____

_____

_____

_____

_____

How do different types of music effect my emotions?

_____

_____

_____

_____

_____

_____

_____

Table of Contents

Before You Begin

SongShine Singing Stars 8

Greetings 12

Personal Acknowledgments 13

I'll Try 17

Prelude 18

How to Use Your Textbook 20

Introduction: *SongShine*—Gaining Vocal Strength.......................... 24

Why Sing? To Do Your Brain A Favor.. 25

I. Posture

Posture: A Firm Foundation 28

Keeping It Noble 29

II. Breath Management

How It Works 34

Your Power Pack 34

Four Stages of Your Power Pack 35

Strength Training for Your Power Pack 36

"Do-Re-Mi" Sing-A-Long.. 40

"Wunderbar" Sing-A-Long 42

III. Vocal Fitness

Vocal Fitness: Become A Vocal Athlete 44

How the Human Voice Works 46

Diction-Articulation-Enunciation: The Competitive Edge 47

Working Out with Diction-Articulation-Enunciation 48

"Yankee Doodle" Sing-A-Long 49

"California, Here I Come" Sing-A-Long 50

Humming: Easy Stretches for the Vocal Athlete............................... 51

Humming Exercises 52

Resonance Exercises with M and N 53

Chim Chim Cher-ee!"   Sing-A-Long... 54

IV. Consonants

Consonants: Springboards for the Vocal Athlete 56

Plosive Consonants: Vocal Training 57

Fricative Consonants: Fabulous Friends.................................. 59

G: The Plosive Consonant with Dual Citizenship 59

Plosive and Fricative Vocalise 60

"Sh-Boom" Sing-A-Long 62

"Supercalifragilisticexpialidocious" Sing-A-Long 63

K: The Friend of the Palate 64

K: Vocalises 65

"Music! Music! Music!" Sounding K-A-Long 66

Approximant Consonants: Adding Vitality 67

"There's No Business Like Show Business" Sing-A-Long.................. 68

V. Vowels

Valuable Vowels 70

Why Vowels Are Valuable.. 70

Pure Vowel Sound.. 71

Pure Vowel Vocalises... 72

"Ja Da, Ja Da" Sing-A-Long 73

Vowel Placement 74

Using Your Brain to Trick and Train 75

Diphthongs 76

Diphthongs: Let Them Falling Away..................................... 77

Vocalises: Avoiding Diphthongs 77

"Goodnight, My Someone" Sing-A-Long 79

VI. Improving Your Skill

Stopping Tone: A Stealth Operation 82

Starting Tone: **H** is for **H**elping Avoid Glottal Fry 83

Vocalises: Avoiding Glottal Fry.. 84

Artistry and Control: Crescendo-Decrescendo-Legato.................... 85

Vocalises: Crescendo-Decrescendo-Legato 85

"Oklahoma"   Sing-A-Long...86

"Edelweiss"   Sing-A-Long 87

VII. Vocal Range Extension

Range Extension 90

Upward Range Extension: The Yawn 90

Vocalises for Upward Range Extension 90

Downward Range Extension: "Buzzzzzzz" 92

VIII. Refining Your Art

Legato: Smooth Flowing Singing 94

Legato Vocalises 94

Adding Agility Requires Flexibility and Precision 96

Agility Vocalises 96

"Climb Ev'ry Mountain"   Sing-A-Long 98

IX. The Wrap Up

Stay in the Game 102

X. Additional Tools

Going to the Vocal Gym SongShine Style 104

Five-Day Vocal Workout...104

Be A Winner: Use the Five-Day Vocal Workout CD 105

Day 1...106

Day 2...108

Day 3...110

Day 4...112

Day 5...114

Addendum

Appendix A: Vocalises for Vocal Ease CD (gold)...............118

Appendix B: SongShine Sing-A-Long CD (blue) 119

Appendix C: Five Day Vocal Workout CD (white) 120

Permissions...121

About the Founder and Author 124

SongShine Singing Stars

by Janet Huff

Sing a song with SongShine,
Sing along with me!
Joyful noise with patience all
for patients with PD.

Don't forget the ones who sang
but years have stripped and 'broke'
the voice that used to sing all day,
Now a whisper – or a croak!

Somehow life just comes along
and knocks away the props!
No longer can we do as much.
So, now we feel like flops!

But never fear, a song is near!
Just come to class and sing!
You may not sing by note or ear,
but glad your heart will ring!

SongShine is for everyone
who feels a hurt, – alas!
You, too, can find a joyful place
in SongShine's happy class!

Come. We welcome everyone,
no matter who you are.
Sing along a SongShine song.
You'll be a SongShine star!

© Janet Huff
July 27, 2010

[dedicated to the founder of SongShine – Ruthanna Metzgar]

8

SongShine Singing Stars

Janet Huff

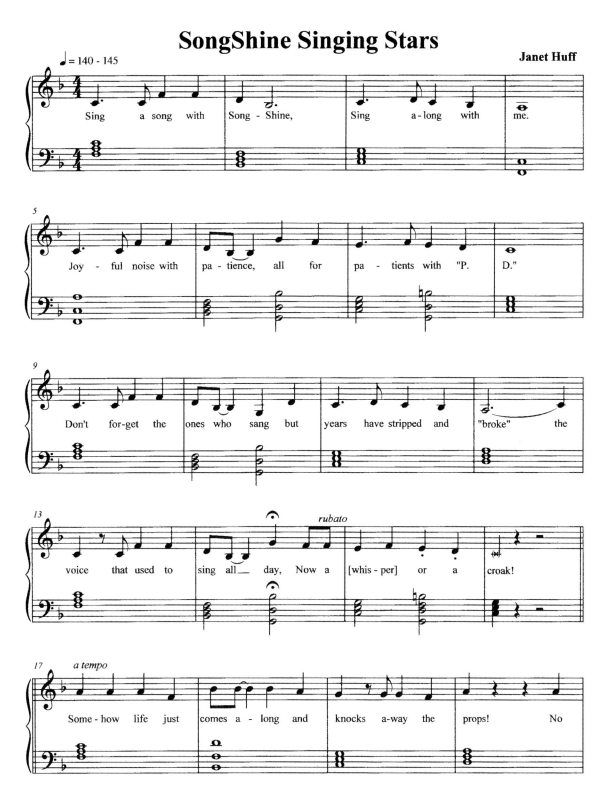

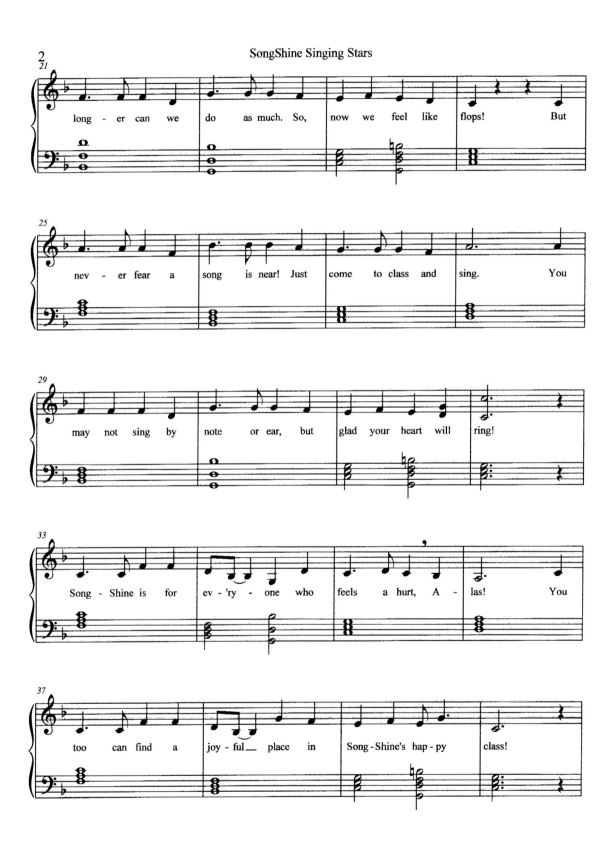

SongShine Singing Stars

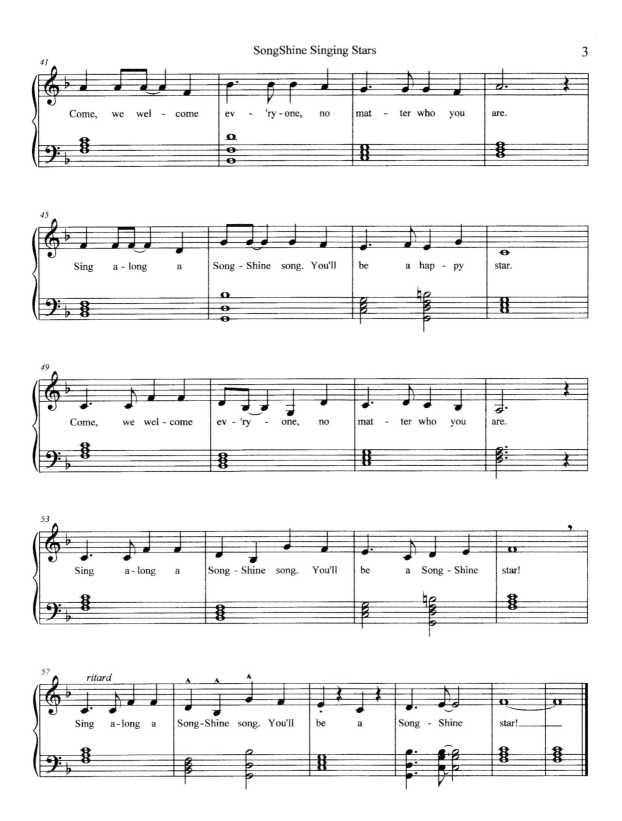

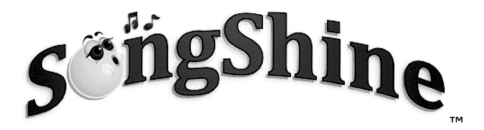

Greetings

SongShine is designed to be a positive learning experience. It is an opportunity to allow music to lift your spirit, touch your heart, release memories, and strengthen your speaking voice. *SongShine* provides a supportive and interactive community created for you.

SongShine is not intended to replace scientifically based traditional medicine, regular visits to your doctor, traditional speech therapy, or physical therapy.

SongShine has developed from information gleaned throughout forty-plus years of teaching voice, reading, working with speech pathologists and otolaryngologists, and exploring ideas with colleagues. I hope that practicing the vocalises, exercises, and songs provided in this textbook will strengthen and improve your vocal health. It is also my hope that being a part of the *SongShine* family will give you a greater appreciation for the joy and healing power of music.

Ruthanna Metzgar, DMA

Founder and Director of SongShine

Acknowledgments

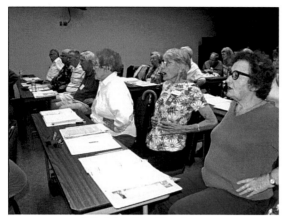
Working hard in class

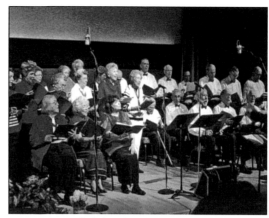
Celebrating in Concert

Special thanks to the class members of *SongShine,* with whom I have been privileged to work during the past four years (2006-2010). As the *SongShine* curricula developed, your enthusiasm and support have challenged me to keep writing, refining and developing my ideas and methods. Your unflagging ability to work hard, share hugs, laugh often, and carry each other's burdens has enriched my life.

Jeannette Debonne, Director of Arts in Healthcare at Eisenhower Medical Center, Rancho Mirage, CA, has been an encourager, friend, and mentor. Thank you, Jeannette, for your adept administrative skill, compassion, support, and dedication to developing the fine arts as a healing modality at Eisenhower Medical Center, Rancho Mirage, CA. Many thanks for making me part of your "tribe."

SongShine could not have survived without Michael Landes, President of the Eisenhower Foundation, Eisenhower Medical Center, Rancho Mirage, CA. Mr. Landes' skillful leadership, compassionate spirit, and clear vision for the healing power of the arts, has kept the department of Arts in Healthcare, of which *SongShine* is a part, alive during turbulent economic times. Thank you, Michael.

My sincere thanks to Traub Parkinson's Center and Susan Hegge, Director of the Center for Healthy Living, Eisenhower Medical Center, Rancho Mirage, CA, whose administrative support and enthusiasm created the initial opportunity for me to develop *SongShine*.

Aaron Green deserves kudos for his superb skill with lighting, sound, and special effects, combined with sensitivity to the needs of class member's during our *SongShine* Celebration Concerts. He has enabled our productions to be smoother and far more professional than we could have ever dreamed. You have made us feel like *SongShine Singing Stars*.

Acknowledgments

To the dedicated and competent support staff at Annenberg Center for Health Sciences on the EMC campus, where classes meet weekly November-April, you are tops.

Special thanks to my extremely skilled classroom assistants, Laurie Tenyecke, music and fine arts teacher, who expertly covers the details of keeping us in the right place, on the right page, at the right time, and Merv Roberts, technical guru *par excellence*, who keeps me wired for sound, my computer working, and graciously lends a hand wherever needed.

It brings me great joy to say *"merci beaucoup"* to my dear friends Joel and Barbara Hochberg. As a film maker, Joel Hochberg has created several wonderful *SongShine* documentaries. His enthusiasm for *SongShine,* passion for filmmaking, and professional skill has given all of us a lasting legacy. You are doing *mitzvah!* And to Barbara, Joel's gracious and talented wife; you deserve many hugs of thanks for your encouragement to our class and to me, personally. The world needs more wonderful people like both of you.

To Ruth Wilkes, master teacher, for her unfailing encouragement and desire to see this project succeed, many thanks for each timely phone call.

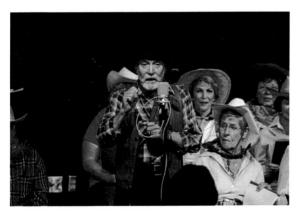

SongShine goes western.

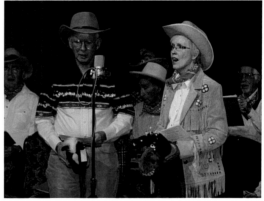

SongShine buckaroos.

Many thanks to Dr. Kenneth Faw, former voice student, and for many years my otolaryngologist, who first piqued my curiosity about the physiological aspects of singing. As he quietly shared his vast knowledge concerning the human voice, he unknowingly started me down this path.

Acknowledgments

To dear neighbors and friends, Ray Jorgensen, MD, Otolaryngology, and his wife Carroll Jorgensen, RN, for enduring numerous phone calls and sudden visits when questions or ideas popped into my head and needed medical verification. Thank you for the many hours and hours spent editing the manuscript. This textbook could not have come into being without your help.

Additionally, there were excellent suggestions and edits from an additional host of dear friends: English teacher Pat Bishop; music educator Jack Bishop; speech pathologists Christine Engelhardt and Martin Nevdahl; journalist and faithful sister Rosemarie Alexander Isett; musician and writer Janet Huff; poetess Nancy Spiellman; linguist William Tang; and music educator, conductor, editor and colleague, Dianne Vars.

The *SongShine* "Sing-A-long" CD of popular songs, was skillfully arranged, played, recorded, and edited by my long-time friend and gifted accompanist, Dorothy Anderson. Dorothy's talent has created an opportunity for all SongShiners to Sing-A-long with style! Thank you, Dorothy.

Finally, had it not been for the patience, mentoring, encouragement, and technical assistance with formatting, I could never have created this document. Thank you, Joe Noegel, for being a dear friend in a time of need.

Any remaining errors or omissions in this document are strictly my own.

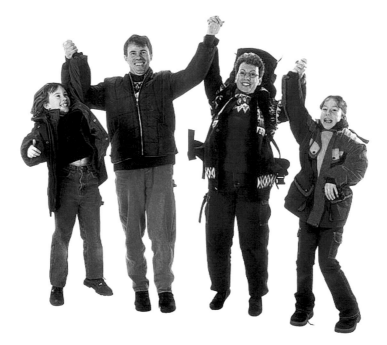

It Took Teamwork!

Special Acknowledgment

SongShine could never have become a reality, or this book written, had it not been for the sacrifices made by my husband, Roy. His vision for its potential came into focus when his cousin, whom he greatly admired, developed Parkinson's.

Throughout the past four years Roy has encouraged, challenged, edited countless pages, listened to hundreds of ideas, forfeited vacations, expended personal finances, washed dishes, done laundry, and vacuumed, all of which freed me to read, write, record, brainstorm, teach, and develop *SongShine.* Perhaps the greatest sacrifice on his part, especially during the summer of 2010, has been setting aside mountaineering adventures together so that I could continue to climb this mountain, and complete the *SongShine* textbook. As with many of our adventures, it has taken teamwork to reach the summit.

ROY, YOU'RE THE BEST!

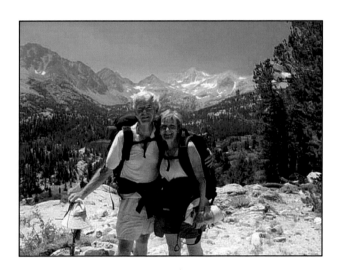

Roy and Ruthanna (2007) hiking in the Sierras.

I'll Try *

Can I, will I give it a try?
Can I, will I be so bold?
Never to give up or fold,
Or am I already too old?

No cause or no cure
Will help me endure.
Could cunning ensure?
What else might assure?

Am I too weary for even a sigh?
Let time pass without even a try?
No, even with closure perhaps nigh,
I'll muster strength for another try.

It seems natural to cry,
But I don't know why.
Will lots of shed tears
Calm anxiety or fears?

If time is running out,
It would be easy to pout.
No, I won't go that route!
I'm ready for another bout!

And if the result
Turns out an insult,
No one should decry
My best efforts to try.

*Dedicated to participants in the inaugural SongShine Program held at the Eisenhower Medical Center, Rancho Mirage, California.

Written August 2010, by Roy G. Metzgar

Prelude

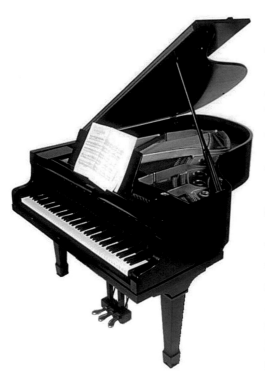

My childhood home nestled in a beautiful forest preserve on the eastern shore of Lake Michigan. On quiet summer evenings I listened to the rhythm of waves softly lapping the beach, accompanied by a whippoorwill's plaintive song—nature's music. During the day a classical radio station filled our house with more beautiful music—symphonies, opera, art songs, German Lieder. Lessons included piano, organ, violin, snare drum, tympani, and voice; they were further augmented by seven exciting summers studying at Interlochen National Music Camp in northern Michigan. Music was a major part of life. No wonder I pursued it as a career, as my father had dreamed.

Dad was a rural pastor with a huge heart for seniors. Usually, Sunday meant a full house for dinner. Our guests might include one with Lou Gehrig's disease, another recovering from a stroke, one using a walker, another with Parkinson's, and there were many widows and widowers. Dad loved them all; they were part of our lives. As a three year old, I accompanied him on visits to elderly who were confined to their homes. We also went to hospitals, retirement homes, and nursing facilities. Thus, I gained an appreciation and deep respect for these wonderful elders who knew how to persevere through tough times.

Decades passed and inevitably I, too, became a senior citizen. My husband and I retired and began wintering in southern California. One day I received a phone call asking if I would consider "doing something with music for the Traub Parkinson's Center at Eisenhower Medical Center in Rancho Mirage, California; perhaps a sing-a-long?" It seemed natural to say, "Yes."

Personal experiences replayed themselves in my mind. As a university voice instructor, I worked with students who stuttered terribly but sang beautifully. My dad had fought a long battle with Alzheimer's, unable to communicate coherently. In spite of his disease, we could walk the halls of the Alzheimer unit together, singing old hymns without him ever missing a word! My mother suffered a stroke and was unable to speak, but hours before her death she and I sang many of her favorite childhood Sunday school songs. Her voice was strong and her diction clear.

I wondered if singing could possibly strengthen a stroke or Parkinson's patient's speaking voice. Could there be an alternate neurological pathway to circumvent the malfunctioning part of the brain? I became convinced of the possibilities and excited about training and strengthening a person's speech through the medium of music. Events and influences from the time of my childhood through university and adult years became the building blocks for a project bigger than I. Studying music's amazing effect on the brain, collecting and writing suitable vocalises, and developing weekly lessons became a new passion, co-equal with teaching and interacting with my wonderful class of *SongShiners*.

There is a familiar story which compares life to a tapestry. From our human perspective, life's events and trials produce the underside of the tapestry with its knots and loose hanging threads. The beautiful picture is on the reverse side, and once-in-a-while Providence allows us to glimpse the upper, beautiful side of the tapestry. For me, the upper side of the weaving is *SongShine.*

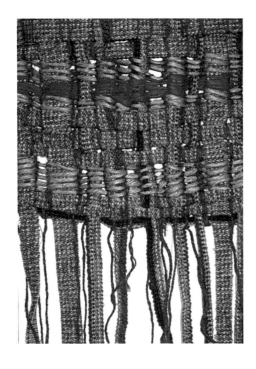
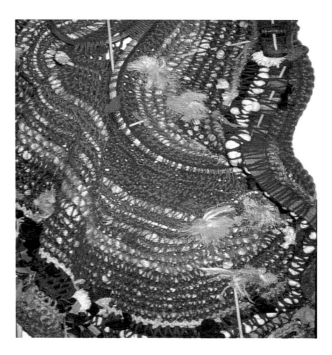

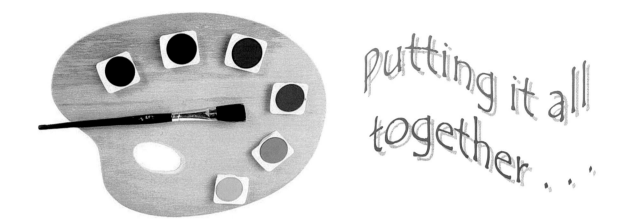

How to Use Your Textbook

Learning to use your textbook will enhance your *SongShine* experience. Your textbook and the CDs included provide the necessary tools to continue improving the quality of your speaking and singing voice on a daily basis.

Table of Contents

The Table of Contents will help you locate everything in the book. It includes all the major topics, sub-topics, and CD information. The Table of Contents is found on page 5 in the textbook.

Text

The text provides information concerning the human voice, posture, breath management, low- or no-impact physical exercises, vocalises, original vocal exercises, lyrics to popular and inspirational songs, and colorful pictures. "Vocalises for Vocal Ease," found in printed form, are scattered throughout. They are arranged according to topic. Near the back of the textbook are five sets of additional vocalises. These are called "Five-Day Vocal Workout." Although all vocal exercises are presented in printed music form, it is not necessary to read music to be able to use this textbook.

Vocalises for Vocal Ease CD (gold)

This CD is a coordinated companion to the printed Vocalises for Vocal Ease in your textbook. Although printed music is provided in the textbook, you do not need to be able to read music to use this CD. Verbal directions are given to make it easy for you to continue practicing all the exercises in the textbook by simply listening and singing along. Having your textbook open as you practice and review your lessons is helpful, but not essential. This CD (gold) is located in the back of your textbook.

Sing-A-Long CD (blue)

Each popular song on this CD coordinates with printed lyrics in your textbook. They have been arranged exclusively for *SongShine* and reinforce techniques learned in class. The selections, written between the 1900s and 1960s, were chosen from standard Broadway, movies, pop, and Americana-type repertoire. Have fun singing along, or simply listening to the music. This CD is located in the back of the textbook.

Five-Day Vocal Workout CD (white)

Five sets of vocalises provide a 15-20 minute vocal workout. Using this CD makes it easy, for those who are serious about staying vocally fit, to practice when not in class. Although printed music for this CD is found in the textbook (see table of contents), you do not need to be able to read music to use this CD. Spoken directions lead you through the CD. The CD is located in the back of your textbook.

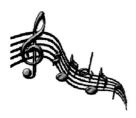

What songs best express . . .

My Dreams:

_____

My Hopes:

_____

My feelings of Patriotism:

_____

My feelings of love:

_____

My feelings of Thanks:

_____

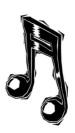

Making it happen . . .

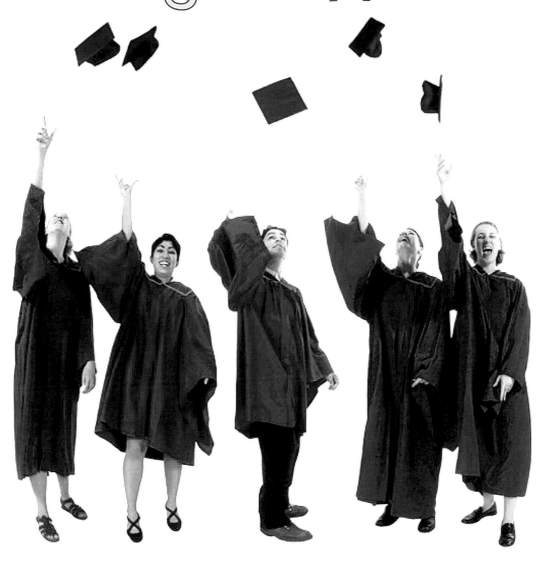

Through the power of music

Introduction

SongShine: **Gaining Vocal Strength**

Through the Power of Music

SongShine is a vocal therapy course designed for persons with Parkinson's disease, stroke, other neurological disorders, or naturally aging voices. Its purpose is to strengthen the speaking voice through exercises called *vocalises* (pronounced vōcal ease).[1] Neurologists understand that speech originates from the left hemisphere of the brain. Research reveals that music is distributed throughout the brain. When the left hemisphere no longer sends strong speech signals, resulting in diminished speech ability, singing allows the speaker to switch channels, to access another pathway. Through vocalises and other original singing exercises, *SongShine* vocal therapy facilitates a retraining or recovery of speech.

Method

Vocalises have been used for centuries by professional singers for the development of a healthy voice. SongShine employs those exercises to gain or restore vocal strength and control. Vocalises improve tone quality, increase vocal range,[2] give agility, build stamina, facilitate diction, and improve mobility of the soft palate. Exercises designed to improve breath management help increase previously underused lung capacity and benefit respiratory function. In addition, students learn how consonants, vowels, and other basic speech components influence the voice. Adding further enjoyment to each class, popular songs are sung to augment vocalises and speech principles being learned. An optional event, a Celebration Concert, is held for participants' families and friends. The concert allows students to demonstrate their progress and share the enjoyment of group and individual accomplishment.

---

[1]*Vocalise* is a French word used to describe a singing exercise used to promote and maintain a beautiful and healthy voice. Correct pronunciation of the plural form, *vocalizes*, requires the final 's' remain silent.

[2] Range: The complete number of pitches, from the highest to the lowest, that one's voice is capable of singing.

Why Sing? To Do Your Brain A Favor

Music is an integral part of our human experience; our planet is awash in it. Although one may not classify all nature's sounds as music, from an academic, intellectual, or humanly organized standpoint, one cannot deny that our brains have processed and learned from the natural musical tones and rhythms around us—nature's music.

Until mechanical noise from the industrial revolution began to compete with natural sound, previous generations were accustomed to living in a world filled with bird song, buzzing insects, wind moaning in the trees, rhythmic horse's hooves, wolves baying at the moon, waves rhythmically crashing onto the beach, or the sounds of waterfalls and creeks. Many of the compositions of such famous classical composers as Bach, Beethoven, Mozart, and Schubert clearly imitate the rhythmic and melodic sequences of quail, nightingale, lark, robin, mockingbird, dove, and cuckoo. Austrian composer, Gustav Mahler, correctly observed, "Man cannot live apart from his surroundings."[3] We are hard-wired for music and nature beckons us to listen and participate.

Listening to music, singing, playing an instrument, dancing or moving in rhythm can soothe or stimulate. An ancient example, chronicling music's soothing power, is found in the Hebrew Scriptures. When torment and anxiety came upon King Saul "…David would take his harp and play. Then relief would come to Saul; he would feel better, and the evil spirit would leave him."[4] From the Baroque Era (1600-1750) music historian Michael Ballam tells us that listening to G. F. Handel's "Water Music" brought King George I relief from headaches caused by stressful matters of state.

Currently, a growing number of hospitals, including the prestigious Mayo Clinic, incorporate live music in hallways, patients' rooms, and post-operative settings; skillfully played calming instruments such as harp or classical guitar are a soothing augmentation to chemical medication.

Musicophilia, by Oliver Sacks, MD,[5] *This is Your Brain on Music,* by Daniel Levintin, PhD,[6] *and The Mozart Effect,* by Don Campbell,[7] each in a unique way chronicle the amazing effects of music on the human brain. As you begin your journey through *SongShine* you may discover some of these wonderful benefits.

---

[3] Knud Martner, ed., trans. Eithne Wilkins, Ernst Kaiser, and Bill Hopkins. *Gustav Mahler: Selected Letters,* 1979, New York; Farrar, Straus, Giroux.

[4] The *Holy Bible,* ISamuel 17:14-23. New International Version. 1984. Grand Rapids:Zondorvan.

[5] Sacks, Oliver, *Musicophillia, Tales of Music and the Brain.* 2008. New York: Vintage Books.

[6] Levintin, Daniel J. *This is Your Brain on Music.* 2007. New York: Plume Books.

[7] Campbell, Don. *The Mozart Effect.* 2001. New York. Harper Collins.

Take time each day to listen, play an instrument, sing, or move rhythmically. Music is powerful. *SongShine* attempts to tap into that power for the purpose of gaining vocal strength. *Why sing? To do your brain and your voice a favor.*

Suggestions

Listen to music from:

Radio, TV, CD, tape, 33 1/3s, 45s, possibly 78s, or your iPod

Move rhythmically to music

Sing

Play an instrument

Dance

Attend a concert

Listen to Nature's Music:

Birds

Crickets

Wind in the trees

A Babbling Brook

Thunder

Squirrels

And One More Musical Sound:

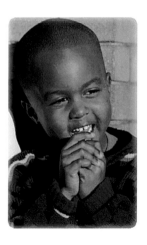

The Laughter of Children

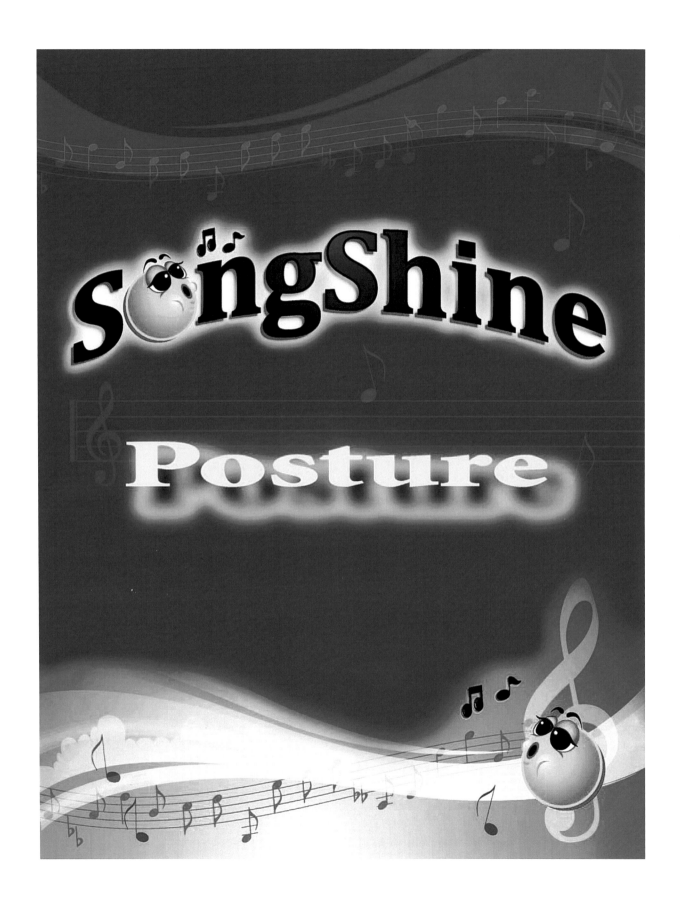

I. Posture: A Firm Foundation

Excellent posture is the foundation of good speaking and singing. It should be relaxed and never tense or rigid. Whether standing or sitting, a person's posture either strengthens or weakens speech and song. Posture can indicate how we are feeling physically, how we feel about ourselves emotionally, and can affect our physical and vocal health.

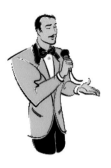

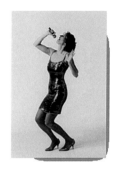

Good Posture

Poor Posture

If standing, place your feet a comfortable distance apart, either parallel to each other or one foot slightly forward. Allow your weight to rest *lightly* on the balls of your feet. Avoid rocking back on your heels or locking your knees. It is important to find a position that makes you feel comfortable and secure as you stand and sing. The boys below appear to have it figured out.

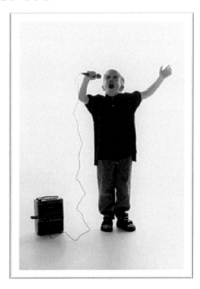

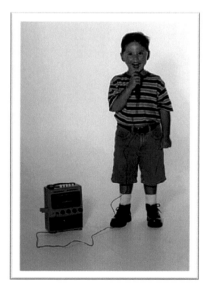

When standing, find the position that makes you feel secure.

If sitting, slide as far back into the chair as possible. The small of your back should touch the back of the chair. Place your feet flat on the floor. If your feet do not touch the floor, slide forward and place a pillow behind your back. Avoid crossing knees or ankles because it can negatively affect the way you breathe and the way you sound. The picture below gives good and bad examples.

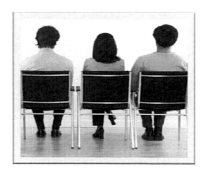

Keeping It Noble

1. Excellent Posture is Noble Posture

Noble posture is that which is stately; simply stretch or lift the mid-section of the body between the navel and the breastbone. Thinking "tall" in this area makes you tall without tension. **Noble posture** is better for the spine, allows the ribs to expand and contract freely, and facilitates deeper breathing.

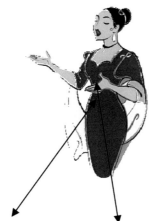

Lifting between the navel and breastbone creates **noble posture**.

2. Noble Posture Means Relaxed Shoulders

When shoulders are relaxed they neither pull upward nor roll forward; both interfere with effective breathing. Try the following for relaxed shoulders.

a. Gently rotate each shoulder (one at a time), making small circles.

b. Using your right hand, gently massage your left shoulder.

c. Using your left hand, gently massage your right shoulder.

d. The distance between your shoulders will look and feel natural as you allow them to relax and assume **noble posture.**

3. Noble Posture Means Relaxed Arms

Whether standing or sitting, excellent posture means your arms are relaxed. Try the following:

a. Gently massage each of your arms with your fingers, moving up and down from the wrist to the shoulder.

b. With your palms facing up, out or down (your choice), raise your arms until they are level with your shoulders. Breathe deeply; as you look at the picture below think of opening your arms to receive the wonders of the world before you.

c. After taking several relaxed breaths, lower your arms to your sides. Allow your fingertips to relax, pointing down-ward; and let your arms hang limp at your sides. If you are sitting, lower your arms and rest your palms on your thighs.

d. Avoid hugging the body with your elbows. Let your arms gently touch the sides of your body.

e. Raise your arms until level with your shoulders; rotate them in large circles. Drop your arms to your sides, allowing your arms to hang as if weightless.

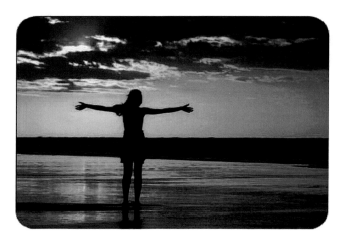

4. Noble Posture Means Relaxed Hands

Our hands can be indicators of relaxation or tension. To relax your hands try the following:

a. Wiggle your fingers for a few seconds.

b. Shake your hands at the wrists.

c. Imagine embracing a large beach ball. Your palms are facing you and fingers are extended toward each other. Slide one hand in front of the other (palms still facing toward you). Make hand circles, moving one hand over the top of the other. Reverse directions.

d. Extend your arms in front of you. With palms down and fingers extended away from your body, make inward and then outward wrist circles.

e. Place your hands at your sides. Take several relaxed slow deep breaths; imagine air is flowing gently into your fingertips.

f. Move your fingers as if playing the piano.

5. Noble Posture Means Relaxed Face, Jaw and Neck

Allowing your face, jaw and neck to relax will help you achieve a more beautiful singing or speaking tone. Combined with **noble posture** you will look and feel more confident. Try the following facial relaxation techniques:

a. Gently massage your temples, cheeks, chin and jaw.

b. Chew in an exaggerated style followed by resting.

c. Open your mouth and stick out your tongue in an exaggerated style as far as you can. Repeat three times.

d. Yawn.

e. Gently massage the back of your neck.

f. Gently nod your head "yes" and "no" several times.

6. Noble Posture Means "Keep a Level Head"

The old adage, "keep a level head," is as important for speaking or singing as it is for life; untrained singers often raise or lower their head or chin trying to "reach" for notes in their upper or lower range. Well trained singers "keep a level head." This does not mean rigidity or the lack of expressive head movement, but rather the absence of "reaching" for notes. Try the following exercise for keeping a level head. If involuntary movement of the head, torso, or limbs makes this exercise difficult, simply focus on the previously presented aspects of **noble posture**.

a. Stand or sit using noble posture.

b. Place a hard-bound book on top of your head.

c. Release your hold on the book.

d. Speak or sing a few words or notes; does the book fall or remain in place?

Remember: the purpose of this exercise is not to create rigidity but to help you establish **noble posture**.

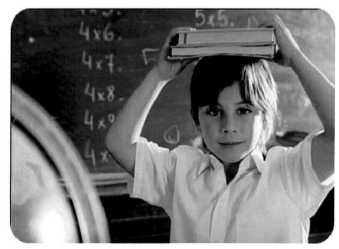

Keep a level head.

7. Noble Posture Means Learning to Relax

Our speaking and singing voices benefit from the absence of tension. Here are a few additional ways to help you relax and relieve tension.

a. Tension is common when trying something new; as noble posture becomes a habit it will add confidence when singing or speaking.

b. Sing as if no one is listening. Have you ever sung in the shower? Close your eyes and pretend you are there as you sing.

c. Visualize a beautiful, peaceful scene; imagine yourself stepping into the scene. Take several deep breaths; open your eyes and smile.

d. Tense your entire body. Hold the tension for three counts. Slowly relax your entire body, from the top of your head clear down to your toes.

e. Listen to a favorite song; gently move or sway to the rhythm.

Noble posture is one of the best friends you can have. Make that friendship second nature. Take **noble posture** with you everywhere you go.

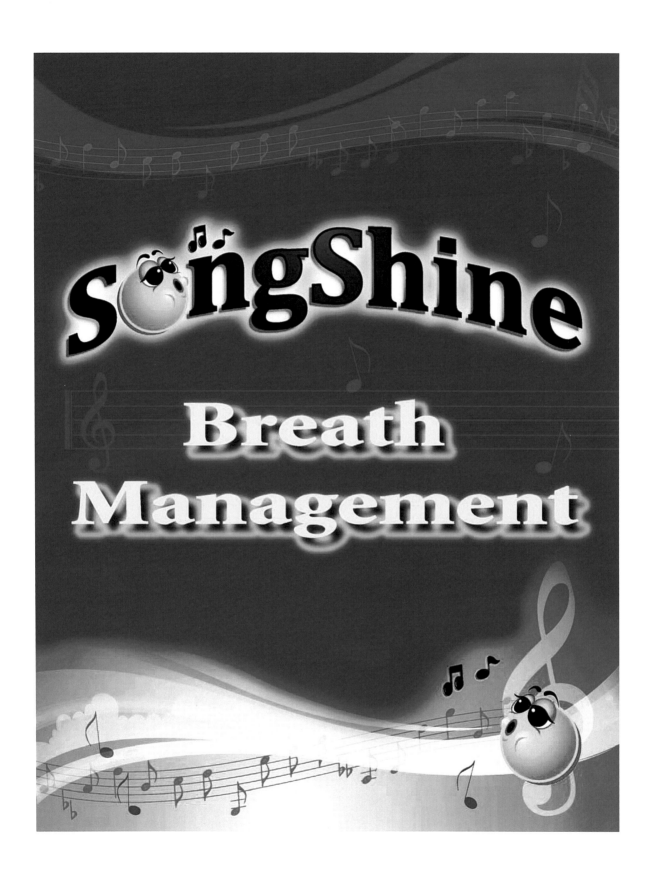

II. Breath Management

Now that you have established **noble posture** your next goal is **breath management**. Most of us breathed perfectly as little babies, especially when crying; but with aging or neurological disorders, breathing often becomes less and less efficient. The lack of lung power is evidenced in decreased vocal sound and changes in voice quality.

How It Works

It is an amazing but simple process: Air (oxygen) is brought into and released from the lungs, which are assisted and protected by the ribs, and activated by muscles. There are two ways to breathe: **Clavicular** or **Diaphragmatic/Costal**.

   1. **Clavicular breathing** is shallow and fills only a small upper portion of the lungs. Unfortunately, older adults are often shallow clavicular breathers.

   2. **Diaphragmatic/costal breathing** fills the upper, middle, and lower portions of the lungs. Singers, wind instrument players, professional speakers, and athletes use this type of breathing.

Think of your lungs as two balloons. Filling balloons with a small amount of air results in small, limp balloons. Filling balloons fully creates greater air pressure on the insides of the balloons, providing more energy (air) available for release. To fully energize the vocal mechanism for healthy speech or song, an adequate amount of air is necessary. As a general rule breathe deeply (low) and slowly rather than rapidly and shallow (high).

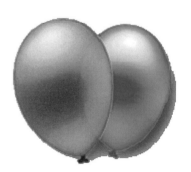

Your Power Pack

A good name for this system of available lung power is **power pack.** Most of us rarely use the power available for speech or song because we fail to breathe deeply and utilize the energy supplied from air—filled lungs. For restoration and maintenance of a healthy voice, a person must use the **power pack** effectively. Filling your **power pack** has additional benefits: a healthier cardio-vascular system, a lower heart rate, stress reduction, and relaxation.

Four Stages of Your Power Pack

There are four stages to healthy breathing for speech and song: **inhalation**, **suspension**, **exhalation**, and **rest**.

1. Inhalation

Inhalation is the act of breathing air deeply into the lungs; it is done either through the nose or mouth. It fills the **power pack** with oxygen/air (energy).

2. Suspension

Suspension occurs when air is suspended for a split second or less immediately following inhalation. The moment suspension occurs, energy (air) from the **power pack** is ready for use in speech or song. This is an automatic process. It happens so quickly you need not concern yourself. Never try to "hold your breath" before you start to sing or speak as it can cause unnecessary tension.

3. Exhalation

Exhalation is the act of releasing air (energy) from the **power pack** (lungs). Exhalation occurs the moment speaking or singing begins. The **power pack** is at work with the vocal folds (cords) to create sound.

4. Rest

Rest occurs the moment sound stops, just before the next breath or inhalation takes place. Momentarily, the **power pack** is empty and ready for refilling.

Many years ago, when all gas stations had service attendants a common expression was "fill it up." That's good advice for speakers and singers, especially those with Parkinson's, stroke or aging voices. When it comes to using your **power pack** efficiently, think "fill it up."

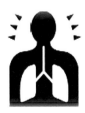 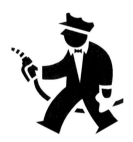

"Fill it up!"

Strength Training for Your Power Pack

The exercises below are designed to help you feel your **power pack** working and strengthen **diaphragmatic/costal breathing.**

1. Ribcage Expansion

    a. Establish noble posture.

    b. Place your hands on the sides of the rib cage, above the waist.

    c. Inhale slowly and deeply. Feel the ribs expand.

    d. Suspend the breath for a split second.

    e. Release the breath. Sense the inward movement of the rib cage but do not let the chest wall collapse.

    f. Rest for a moment and repeat several times.

The sketch below shows a side view of the rib cage before a breath (dotted lines) and after a breath (solid lines). It also indicates the area of lift for **noble posture.**

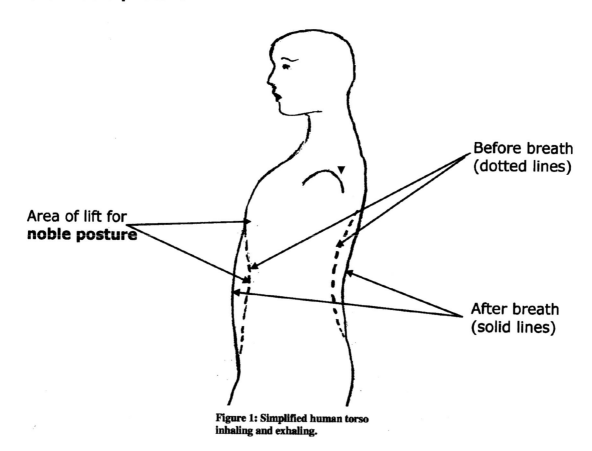

Before breath
(dotted lines)

Area of lift for
noble posture

After breath
(solid lines)

Figure 1: Simplified human torso inhaling and exhaling.

2. Panting Like a Dog

a. Place the palms of your hands flat on your upper-abdominals and allow your middle fingertips to touch; this area of the torso is called the epigastrium.[8] Internally, an unopposed muscle called the diaphragm[9] will move downward as your lungs fill: You will not feel this happen.

b. Open your mouth and pant like a dog, first pant slowly and then pant rapidly. Notice the mid-abdominals moving in and out Warning: Doing this for too long a time may cause dizziness.

3. Drinking Straw

a. Place one end of a drinking straw between your lips.

b. Slowly draw air through the straw. Do you feel the expansion of ribs and abdominals?

c. Suspend the breath for a second.

d. Exhale slowly through the straw. Although your ribcage will move inward as you expel the air, do not allow the chest wall to collapse.

4. Puff on Voiceless "Puh" inhaling at arrows. ⇩

a. Create voiceless puffs on "puh"⇩ "puh" ⇩"puh".

b. Notice the movement of the mid-abdominals.

5. Blow Out the Candle

a. Inhale deeply; allow the ribcage to expand.

b. Blow out the candle using a long, steady stream of air.

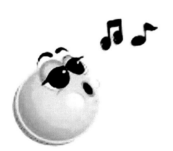 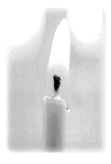

Did the candle go out? ☺

---

[8] The epigastrium is the area of the torso above the navel and below the breast bone.

[9] The diaphragm is an unopposed muscle which separates lungs and viscera. As the lungs fill with oxygen the diaphragm moves downward and allows the lungs to expand. Current emphasis on maintaining a flat, hard, belly will not allow the diaphragm to move through its full range of motion, thus inhibiting maximum breath intake.

6. Hissing at the Clock (Like a Snake)

    a. Watch the second hand on a clock. Inhale deeply and suspend the breath for a second.

    b. Hiss, like a snake. Release a controlled, steady stream of air.

    c. How many seconds can you continue the hissing sound? As you practice (several times a day), the length of time should increase.

7. Hissing in rhythm while clapping.

    a. Make *one* long hissing sound as you clap 1-2-3-4.

    b. Make *two* long hissing sounds (on 1 and 3) as you clap1-2-3-4.

    c. Make *four* hissing pulsations, one on each clap: 1-2-3-4.

    d. Make *eight* short hissing pulsations while clapping 1 & 2 & 3 & 4 &.

    e. Make *sixteen* hissing pulsations while clapping 1-e- &-ah-2-e-&-ah 3-e-&-ah-4-e-&-ah. (Repeat the exercise)

Vocalises for Vocal Ease CD (gold) is a companion to this textbook. Use it to practice the vocalises provided in the text. Reading music is not a requirement; simply listen and sing along.

8. Sing S for Energized Sound.

Vocalises for Vocal Ease CD (gold) Track # 1: Introduction.

Track # 2: Exercises a. and b. as seen below. All are in common time.

    a.

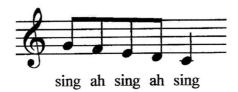

sing ah sing ah sing

    b.

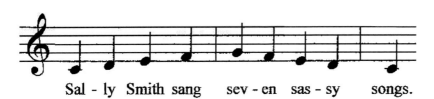

Sal - ly Smith sang sev - en sas - sy songs.

9. Counting Out Loud

a. Inhale deeply; suspend the breath for a second.

b. Slowly count out loud (1..2..3..4..5..6..7..8..9..etc). How far can you count on one breath? Try counting further with each attempt. Remember: noble posture, engage your power pack.

10. Vocalises for Vocal Ease CD (gold) track # 3.

Breathe only at the arrow as you sing the numbers below.

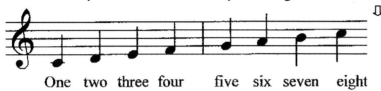

One two three four   five six seven eight

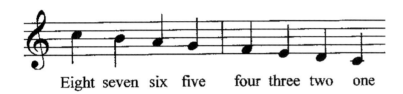

Eight seven six five   four three two one

11. Speaking the Alphabet

a. Inhale deeply and suspend for a second.

b. Speak the alphabet. How many times can you repeat the alphabet in one exhalation? Practice will help you increase the   number of times per exhalation.

c. For a brain teaser, try saying the alphabet backwards.

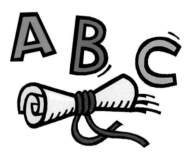

12. Do Re Mi

a. Speak the Italian names of the scale:

Do Re Mi Fa So La Ti Do.

(pronunciation)

 Doh   Reh   Mee   Fah   Soh Lah Tee   Doh

b. Speak them backwards: Do Ti La So Fa Mi Re Do

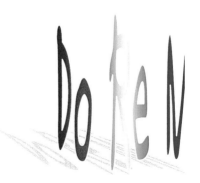

13. Vocalises for Vocal Ease CD (gold) track # 4.

Sing the *Italian* names of the scale, breathing only at the arrow.   ⇩

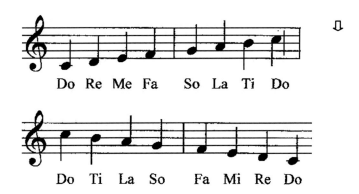

Do Re Me Fa So La Ti Do

Do Ti La So Fa Mi Re Do

Time to Sing-A-Long

Sing-A-Long CD (blue) track #1

Remember **Noble posture**. Engage your **power pack**. Can you sing each line using only one breath?

"Do-Re-Mi"

Doe – a deer, a female deer,
Ray – a drop of golden sun,
Me – a name I call myself,
Far – a long, long way to run,
Sew – a needle pulling thread,
La – a note to follow sew
Tea – a drink with jam and bread.
That will bring us back to do! Oh, oh, oh.

Doe – a deer, a female deer,
Ray – a drop of golden sun,
Me – a name I call myself,
Far – a long, long way to run,
Sew – a needle pulling thread,
La – a note to follow sew
Tea – a drink with jam and bread.
That will bring us back to do!
Do-re-mi-fa-so-la-ti-do.

14. "Surprise!" Smell the Roses.

a. Inhale quickly through the mouth as if you are "surprised". Notice how the soft palate rises. Exhale, but don't let the chest fall.

b. After your "surprise" inhalation, suspend the breath for a second and exhale slowly.

c. Pretend you have a fragrant rose in your hand. Smell the rose. Notice how your rib cage expands. Exhale, keeping noble posture.

15. Yawning

a. Think about yawning and you probably will! As you yawn, notice that air/oxygen enters your lungs, the soft palate rises, and your rib cage expands.

b. Repeat.

16. Floor and Book

This exercise should be done only if you are able to safely get down onto and up from the floor.

a. Lie flat on your back, pressing your spinal column against the floor. Don't arch your back.

b. Lay a medium sized hard-bound book on your mid-abdominals.

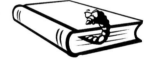

c. Breathe deeply.

d. Notice the book rising and falling as you breathe.

17. Book Exercise: Flexing the Abdominals (Sitting or Standing)

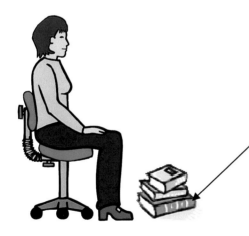

a. Sit or stand tall.

b. Select a hard-bound book and place the book spine against your mid-abdominals.

c. Inhale slowly while holding the book in place.

d. Notice the book moving outward.

e. Suspend the breath for a second.

f. Exhale, noticing the book moving inward.

18. Arm Stretch

a. While sitting or standing, raise your arms to the side until they are level with your shoulders.

b. Inhale and notice ribcage and middle abdominal expansion.

c. Raise your arms straight up. Reach as high as possible. Inhale. Notice the expansion of your ribs, both side and back.

Time to Sing-A-Long

Sing-A-Long CD (blue) track # 2

Employ noble posture and engage your **power pack** as you sing this graceful waltz by Cole Porter. The German word "Wunderbar" means "wonderful". **W** is pronounced like **V**.

"Wunderbar"

Wunderbar, wunderbar! What a perfect night for love,

Here am I, here you are, Why, it's truly wunderbar!

Wunderbar, wunderbar! We're alone and hand in glove,

Not a cloud near or far, Why, it's more than wunderbar!

Oh, I care, dear, for you madly,

And I long, dear, for your kiss.

I would die, dear, for you gladly,

You're divine, dear! And you're mine dear.

Wunderbar, wunderbar! There's our fav'rite star above,

What a bright shining star, Like our love it's Wunderbar!

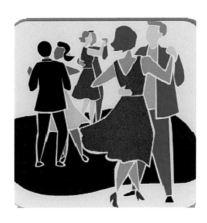

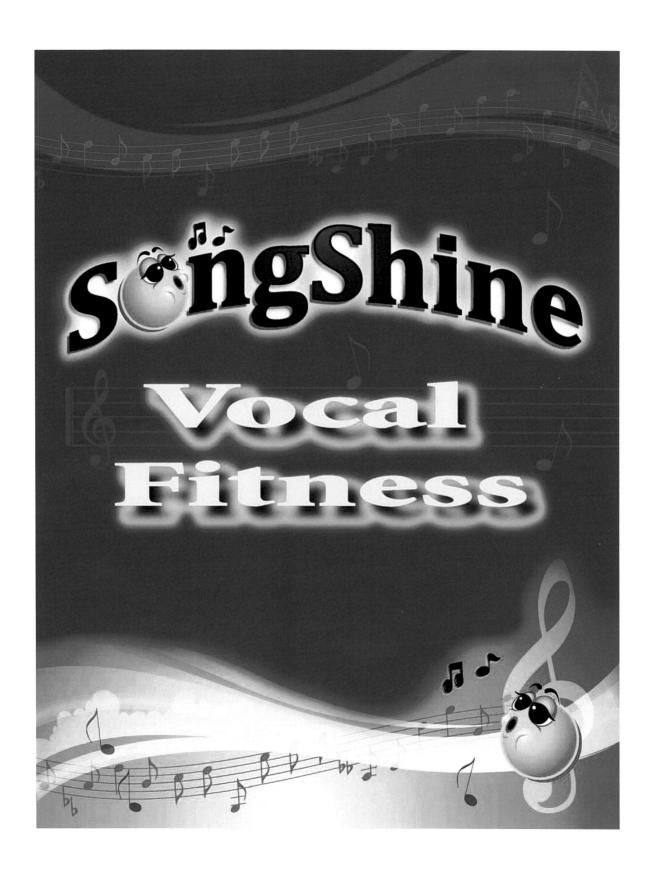

III. Vocal Fitness: Become a Vocal Athlete

Now that you have established noble posture and understand the basic concept of power pack, you need to develop a regimen of vocal fitness to build, regain, and maintain a healthy speaking and singing voice. Become a vocal athlete. There is much we can learn from the athlete's regimen. An athlete's body is carefully prepared for the sport. It would be foolish for a football player to suit up for a game without lifting weights, running, stretching, throwing and catching a ball, and understanding the assigned plays for his position.

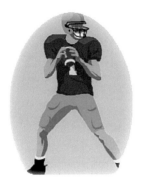 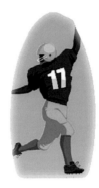 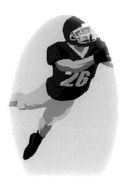

Athletes need to prepare and understand the game.

A gymnast would never attempt the graceful and amazing routines of the sport without preparation: strength training, perfecting balance, stretching muscles, ligaments and tendons, and memorizing the complex routines to be performed. The same applies to a singer.

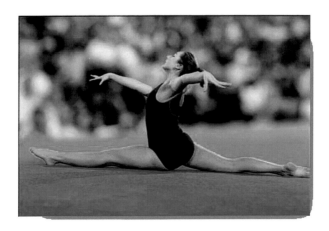

An athlete must be prepared for the routine.

Unless a person is a professional singer or speaker, he or she probably has not considered vocal fitness as part of a daily routine—which is a key to vocal health. When we speak or sing, demands are placed on the voice. Becoming a vocal athlete by staying vocally fit helps you meet those demands. Maintaining a healthy vocal regimen will add strength, stamina and beauty to your voice. Your SongShine textbook includes vocalises and popular songs to make this vocal practice more enjoyable and keep you in the communication game.

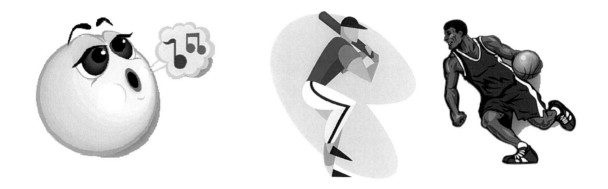

Incorporating music into our daily lives can have positive effects. "Through studies of people with brain damage, we've seen patients who have lost the ability to read a newspaper but can still read music, or individuals who can play the piano but lack the motor coordination to button their own sweater. Music listening, performance, and composition engage nearly every area of the brain that we have so far identified, and involve nearly every neural subsystem. Could this fact account for claims that music listening exercises other parts of our minds; that listening to Mozart twenty minutes a day will make us smarter?"[10] **Become a vocal athlete: it's a smart move.**

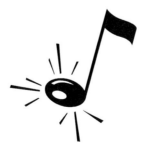

---

[10] *This Is Your Brain On Music,* Daniel J. Levitin. New York. Plume/Penguin Group 2006, pg. 9

How the Human Voice Works

A fine athlete understands his body; knowing muscles, ligaments, tendons, and how they respond to specific exercises and workout regimens adds strength, agility, endurance and grace to the athlete's art. If we are to become a skilled and artful **vocal athlete** we will also benefit from understanding how the voice works. The sketch below provides some basic information.

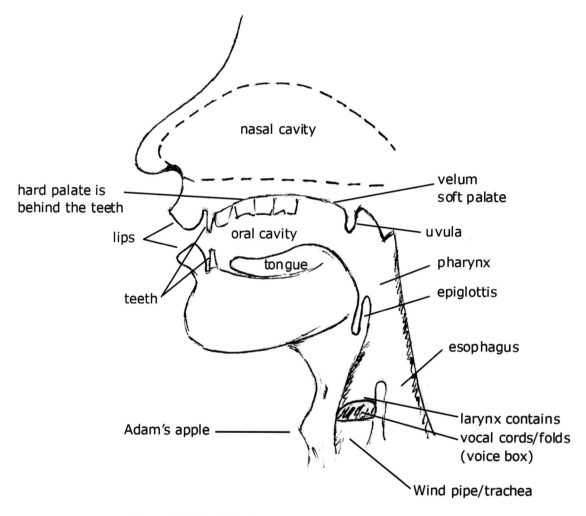

Figure 2: Simplified cross section of human head.

The **larynx** is part of the breathing or respiratory tract which allows us to produce vocal sound. By placing your fingers on your **Adam's apple** and humming or speaking you will feel the vibration of your **vocal chords.** The **vocal cords**, also known as **vocal folds**, are two pieces of flesh capable of being tightened or loosened. When breathing, air flows to and from the lungs and passes freely through open vocal cords. When swallowing, the vocal cords come together and the epiglottis folds back closing the entrance to the wind pipe, which prevents choking. Simultaneously, the velum (soft palate) closes the nasal cavity, preventing food and liquid from escaping through the nose while swallowing.

When singing or speaking, air pressure from the lungs causes the vocal cords to vibrate, creating vocal sound. When we whisper, the cords do not vibrate. The tongue, velum, lips, and oral cavity can change shape and position, creating the variety of consonant and vowel sounds in human speech. The coordination of motor movement and breath is essential for intelligible speech. Each part of the mechanism has a vital and unique role to play in the communication game.

Diction-Articulation-Enunciation: The Competitive Edge

SongShine approaches "speech through song" and "song through speech." An old saying of unknown origin sums it up this way: "Well spoken is half sung." As we have already learned, speaking and singing require oxygen-filled lungs. But having all the breath in the world to energize the power pack would leave us only "full of hot air," as the old saying goes, if it were not for diction, articulation and enunciation. In athletic terms, one might say they give the speaker and singer a competitive edge. The American College Dictionary gives the following definitions:

Diction: "…the degree of distinctness with which speech sounds are Uttered." This means the overall clarity with which we speak.

Articulation: "…the adjustments and movements of speech organs involved in pronouncing a particular sound." This means it is important to retain or regain the ability to move our lips, tongue, jaw, and soft palate in order to maintain clear speech. **Articulation** requires flexibility of the face, jaw and tongue. Parkinson's, stroke, and aging often leave our faces with less flexibility. Regaining flexibility will greatly improve our speech.

Enunciation: "…to utter or pronounce words in a particular manner: *he enunciates his words distinctly.*" This means a better quality of life for those with aging voices, Parkinson's, or speech related stroke issues; others will understand you when you **enunciate** distinctly.

Working Out With Diction-Articulation-Enunciation

Below are ideas for practicing diction, articulation and enunciation. Can you think of other ways to practice clear speech?

1. Read part of your daily newspaper aloud.

2. Read a bedtime story to your grandchildren.

3. Invite friends over to read their favorite poetry aloud.

4. Read a book with a friend, taking turns reading aloud.

5. Sing vocalises and songs every day.

6. Always breathe intentionally before you speak.

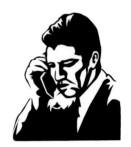

7. Make it a point to call a friend each day, even   if only to say, "I am thinking of you and I am   calling to say, 'have a wonderful day.' " Their day will be brighter and you will have had an opportunity to practice diction, articulation, and enunciation.

8. Try speaking a few of the tongue twisters   below. Speed is not as important as clarity.

- "Peter Piper picked a peck of pickled peppers."

- "She sells sea shells at the seashore."

- "Papa, Papa, picked a peck of peas."

- "If Sue chooses to chew her shoes should she allow Stu to choose the shoes he chews?"

- "How many cookies could a good cook cook if a good cook could cook cookies?."

- "Toy boat, toy boat, floating on the stream remote."

- "This is a thistle and this is a fine vine."

- "Quiet Cape Cod is crammed with colorful quaint cozy cottages."

- "Gentians and geraniums generally bloom jubilantly in June."

- "Bill, Bob, Brandon, and Burt bought brand new basketballs."

- "How many clams can a clam digger cram into a carefully cleaned canning clam can?"

Time to Sing-A-Long

Sing-A-Long CD (blue) track # 3.

Test your ability to **articulate** and **enunciate** using excellent **diction** as you sing this Revolutionary War (1775-1783) song.

"Yankee Doodle"

Father and I went down to camp along with Captain Goodin'
And there we saw the men and boys as thick as hasty puddin'.
Yankee Doodle keep it up, Yankee Doodle dandy,
Mind the music and the step, and with the girls be handy.

And there we saw a thousand men, as rich as Squire David,
And what they wasted every day I wish it could be sav-ed.
Yankee Doodle keep it up, Yankee Doodle dandy,
Mind the music and the step, and with the girls be handy.

And there was Captain Washington upon a slapping stallion,
A-giving orders to his men, I guess there was a million.
Yankee Doodle keep it up, Yankee Doodle dandy,
Mind the music and the step, and with the girls be handy.

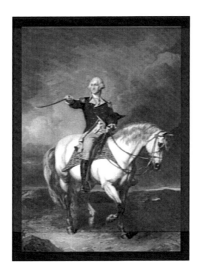

"And there was Captain Washington upon a slapping stallion."

SongShine Sing-A-Long CD (blue) track # 4.

The lively, toe tapping 1924 song, "California, Here I Come," gives us another opportunity to practice excellent diction. Remember: **noble posture**, fill the **power pack**, and most of all—enjoy!

"California Here I Come"

California here I come, right back where I started from.

Where bowers of flowers bloom in the sun,

Each morning at dawning birdies sing and everything.

A sun kissed maid said "don't be late",

That's why I can hardly wait, so, open up your Golden Gate,

California here I come.

California here I come, right back where I started from.

Where bowers of flowers bloom in the sun,

Each morning at dawning birdies sing and everything.

A sun kissed maid said "don't be late", that's why I can hardly wait, so, open up your Golden Gate,

California here I come.

California here I come.

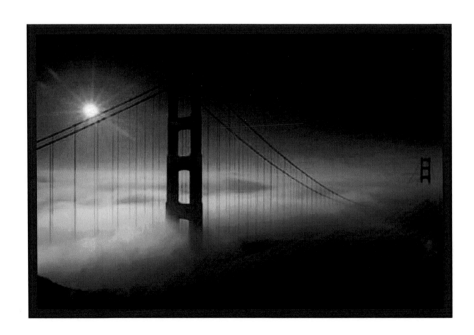

"...so open up your Golden Gate, California, here I come."

Humming: Easy Stretches for the Vocal Athlete

Just as an athlete's routine begins with easy stretching, likewise the singer's routine begins with humming.

Humming is defined as:

1. "Sound which is created without opening the lips…"
2. "A tune which is sung without words or opening the lips…"
3. "To emit a continuous droning sound of an insect on the wing…"
4. "Used to express surprise or displeasure…"
5. "Continuous drone such as a truck, tractor, motor boat…" [11]

Make the following humming sounds without opening your lips:

1. Imitate a mosquito or bumble bee.
2. Express your delight with the taste of your favorite food.
4. Imitate the sound of a motor boat as it skims across the water.
3. Hum a few bars of your favorite tune.

For a Healthy Hum:

1. Imagine having a drop of water between your lips; pressing too hard will cause the water to squirt out and having too much space between the lips will cause the water to dribble out.

2. *Gently* bring your lips together.

3. Select a pitch in the middle of your range—neither too high nor too low. Start humming.

Humming is only the beginning:

It is an important step in developing a vibrant, healthy tone in your singing voice. Try the following exercise:

1. Place the palm of your hand in front of your face an inch or two from your lips and take a breath.

2. Take a deep breath and say the word "hum". Pronounce plenty of **h** to get the breath flowing. Elongate "mmmmmmm".

Healthy humming requires: 1) consistent breath flow, 2) **noble posture**, 3) relaxed facial muscles.

---

[11] *The American Heritage Dictionary of the English Language,* New York, American Heritage Publishing Co., Inc. 1969, p. 640

Humming Exercises

Vocalises for Vocal Ease CD (gold) track # 5.

Begin your vocal warm up with easy stretches.

1.

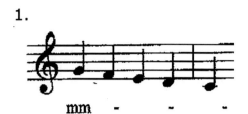

mm -   -   -

2.

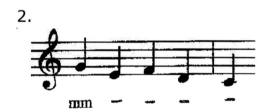

mm -   -   -   -

3.

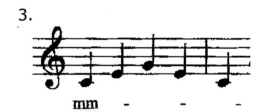

mm -   -   -

Another important sound for warming the voice is created using the letter *n*. Speak the following **n** exercises elongating the **n**. You should feel a vibrating or tingling sensation created just behind the nose:

   1. Nee   Nay   Nah   Noh   Noo

   2. Ned never knew Nelson's nickname.

It is important to learn a variety of exercises that incorporate the letters m and n. These consonants help develop a bright and resonant sound whether speaking or singing. Try making humming sounds when you first awake. It will give your voice a good start with easy stretches.

Resonance Exercises With M and N

Vocalises for Vocal Ease CD (gold) track # 6.

Resonance exercises using **m** or **n** will help build a healthy, vibrant tone. You may substitute **m** or **n** as the beginning letter for the exercises below.

1.

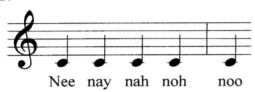

Nee nay nah noh noo

2.

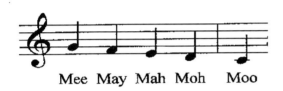

Mee May Mah Moh Moo

3.

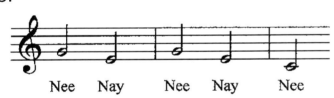

Nee Nay Nee Nay Nee

4.

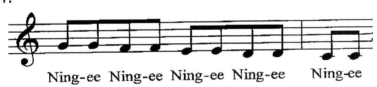

Ning-ee Ning-ee Ning-ee Ning-ee Ning-ee

5.

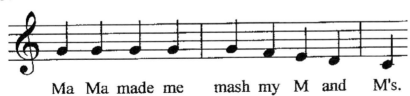

Ma Ma made me mash my M and M's.

6.

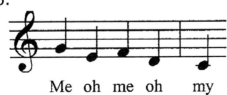

Me oh me oh my

Time To Sing-A-Long

SongShine Sing-A-Long CD (blue) track # 5

In the 1964 Disney movie, _Mary Poppins,_ Bert sang about his life above the London roof tops as a chimney sweep. "Chim, Chim, Cher-ee," offers lots of practice on **m** and **n**.

"Chim Chim Cher-ee"

Chim Chim-in-ey, chim chim-in-ey
Chim chim cher-ee!
A sweep is as lucky as lucky can be.
Chim Chim-in-ey, chim chim-in-ey
Chim chim cher-oo!
Good luck will rub off when I shakes 'ands with you,
Or blow me a kiss and that's lucky too!

Up where the smoke is all billered and curled,
'Tween pavement and stars,
is the chimney sweep world.
When there's 'ardly no day nor 'ardly no night,
There's things 'alf in shadow and 'alf-way in light
On the roof tops of London, Coo what a sight!

Chim Chim-in-ey, chim chim-in-ey
Chim chim cher-ee!
When you're with a sweep you're in
glad company.
Nowhere is there a more 'appier crew
Than them wot sings,
Chim chim cher-ee, chim cher-oo!
Chim Chim-in-ey chim chim, cher-ee, chim cher-roo!

Don't lose your balance way up there! ☺

Singing each day will speed you on your way to becoming a **vocal athlete**. In addition to strengthening the speaking voice, there are other benefits: According to music therapist Donalyn Richardson, there is a reason many of us like to sing in the shower; it seems to make us feel good.

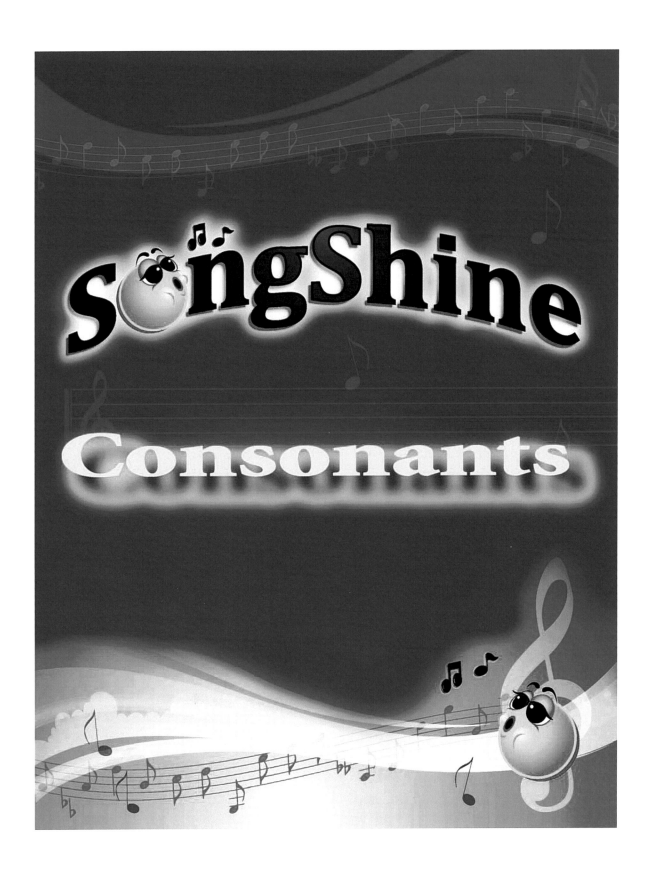

IV. Consonants: Springboards for Vocal Athletes

The diver is being propelled upward by the energy, lift, and buoyancy provided by the action of the springboard.

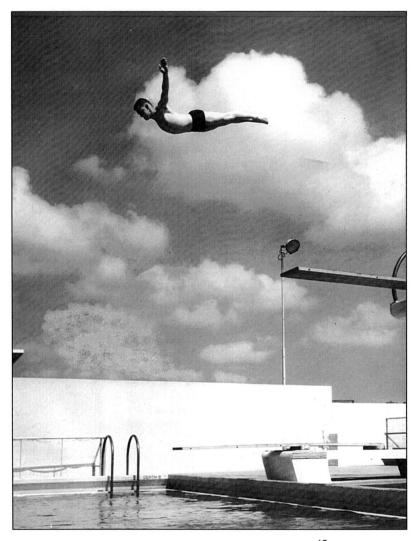

The board gives energy and lift...[12]

Consonants have a similar effect in speech and song. They are springboards which energize the voice. Consonants propel the sound forward, giving energy, direction, and clarity to speech. There are three basic types of consonants: **plosives, fricatives,** and **approximants**.

---

[12] Photo used by permission.

Plosive Consonants: Vocal Strength Training

Plosive consonants, also called "stopped" consonants, are those in which air is stopped momentarily and then "explodes" when released. **Plosive consonants** are an important component of healthy speech and song. They give power, energy, and thrust to words. Although there are many classifications of plosives, for our purposes, we will focus simply on their benefit as great energizers of sound.

 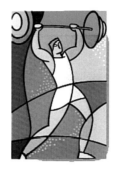 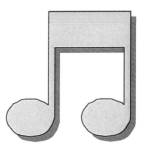

1. Speak the **names** of the following **plosive consonants** and notice the explosion of air.

K	P	B	T	D

2. Speak the ***sound*** of each letter. You will notice that the "sound" is different than the actual "letter name". Although there are reasons for this, for our purposes the important thing is to notice the explosion of air.

K	P	B	T	D

3. Sing each of the following sequences on any comfortable mid-range pitch. Notice the energy a **plosive consonant** creates at the beginning of each syllable: a verbal springboard propelling tone forward.

KEE	KAY	KAH	KOH	KOO
PEA	PAY	PAH	POH	POO
BEE	BAY	BAH	BOH	BOO
TEA	TAY	TAH	TOH	TOO
DEE	DAY	DAH	DOH	DOO

4. The following words have **plosives** at both ends. Notice the beginning and ending "explosion."   Use your **power pack**—it's dynamite!

Keep   Pack   Tube   Duck   Tick   Peak   Book   Take   Bib

5. Exaggerate the **plosives** as you slowly sing the exercise below. Notice the energy in the sound. Take a breath after each word.

Vocalises for Vocal Ease CD (gold) track # 7.

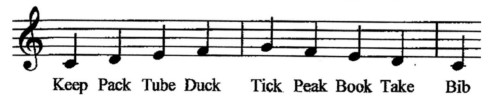

Keep Pack Tube Duck   Tick Peak Book Take   Bib

Plosive consonants are excellent for building strength and energy into the voice. They are building blocks for becoming a **vocal athlete**. Whether speaking or singing, **plosives** are energizers.

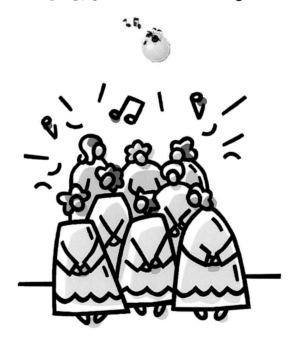

"I hear plosives in the air, they're exploding everywhere."

Fricative Consonants: Fabulous Friends

Fricative Consonants "impede" or create "friction" as air flows through or over the tongue, lips, or teeth. Like **plosives**, they energize speech. There are two types of **fricatives**, "voiced" or "voiceless". **Voiced fricatives** allow the vocal cords to vibrate, as in normal speech. **Voiceless fricatives** are like whispering; the vocal cords do not vibrate. As you speak each bolded letter and word below, "feel" the subtle differences and sensations created by both types of **fricatives**.

f	**fine**	voiceless
v	**vine**	voiced
th	**thistle**	voiceless
th	**this**	voiced
s	**sue**	voiceless
z	**zoo**	voiced
sh	**shore**	voiceless
ch	**chore**	voiceless
z	**azure**	voiced
sh	**assure**	voiceless

Create the sounds of the voiceless fricatives below. This is **"The Waltz of the Voiceless Fricatives."**

F	**CH**	**CH**		**SH**	**S**	**S**		**TH**	**TH**	**CH**	**F** **S** **S**
SH	**F**	**F**		**CH**	**SH**	**SH**		**S**	**S**	**TH**	**CH** **F** **F**

G: The Plosive Consonant With Dual Citizenship

The consonant **G** can function as either a **fricative** or **plosive**. When it is found in words like "gate" or "good," it is a **plosive**. But when you say "hello" to "Gerry" or "George" it is a **fricative**. It is a little like holding "dual citizenship." ☺

When vocal power is diminished by Parkinson's, Stroke, or aging, practicing **fricatives** and **plosives** helps strengthen speech and song. Like runners needing an extra burst of energy, **fricatives** and **plosives** energize sound. These are fabulous friends because they help singers and speakers "cross the finish line."

Plosive and Fricative Vocalises

Vocalises for Vocal Ease CD (gold) track # 8
Sing the following **plosive and fricative** vocalises.
Check: Is your posture **noble** and your **power pack** engaged?

1.
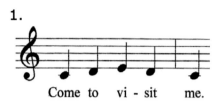
Come to vi - sit me.

2.
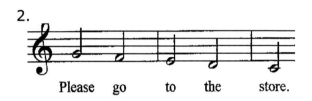
Please go to the store.

3.
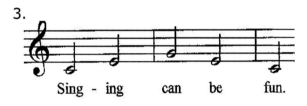
Sing - ing can be fun.

4.
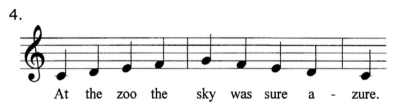
At the zoo the sky was sure a - zure.

5.
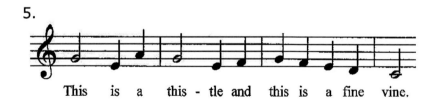
This is a this - tle and this is a fine vine.

6.

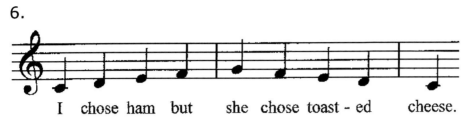

I chose ham but she chose toast - ed cheese.

7.

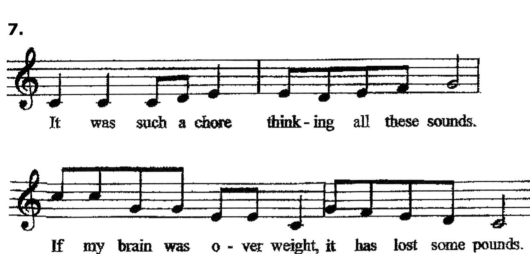

It was such a chore think - ing all these sounds.

If my brain was o - ver weight, it has lost some pounds.

Practicing vocal exercises daily will add strength to your voice and clarity to your diction. Just as athletes have a daily routine for keeping fit, likewise **vocal athletes** need a daily routine for keeping their voices in top condition. Vocalises are like taking vitamins for your voice. When challenged by age or neurological disorders, maintaining a healthy routine of exercise and vitamins is a win—win, whether for the body or the voice.

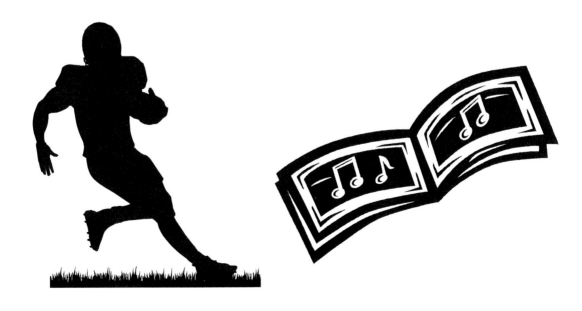

Time to Sing-A-Long

Sing-A-Long CD (blue) track # 6.

Considered the first real *doo wop* song of the 1950's, "Sh-Boom" is a **plosive** and **fricative** workout.

"Sh-Boom"

Sh-boom,   sh-boom
Ya-da-da   da-da-da   da-da-da   da
Sh-boom,   Sh-boom
Ya-da-da   da-da-da   da-da-da da
Sh-boom,   Sh-boom
Ya-da-da   da-da-da   da-da-da   da
Sh-boom!

Life could be a dream-,
If I could take you up in Paradise up above-,
If you would tell me I'm the only one that you love,
Life could be a dream, sweetheart.
Hel-lo, hel-lo again,
Sh-boom, and hope-in' we'll meet again.

Oh, life could be a dream-,
If only all my precious plans would all come true-,
If you would let me spend my whole life lovin' you,
Life could be a dream, sweetheart.

Sh-boom,   sh-boom
Ya-da-da   da-da-da   da-da-da   da
Sh-boom,   Sh-boom
Ya-da-da da-da-da   da-da-da da
Sh-boom,   Sh-boom
Ya-da-da   da-da-da   da-da-da   da
Sh- boom!

Life could be a dream, sweetheart.
Life could be a dream, sweetheart.

Sing-A-Long CD (blue) track # 7.

Here is another "super" song for practicing **fricatives** and **plosives**.

"Supercalifragilisticexpialidocious"

Um diddle diddle diddle, um diddle ay!
Um diddle diddle diddle um diddle ay!

Sup-er-cal-i-frag-il-is-tic-ex-pi-al-i-do-cious!
Even though the sound of it is something quite a-tro-cious!
If you say it loud enough, you'll always sound pre-co-cious.
Su-per-cal-i-frag-il-is-tic-ex-pi-al-i-do-cious!

Um diddle diddle diddle, um diddle ay!
Um diddle diddle diddle, um diddle ay!

Because I was afraid to speak when I was just a lad,
Me father gave me nose a tweak And told me I was bad.
But then one day I learned a word that saved me achin' nose
The biggest word you ever heard and this is how it goes:

Su-per-cal-i-frag-il-is-tic-ex-pi-al-i-do-cious!
Even though the sound of it is something quite a-tro-cious,
If you say it loud enough, you'll always sound pre-co-cious!
Su-per-cal-i-frag-il-is-tic-ex-pi-al-i-do-cious!

Um diddle diddle diddle, um diddle ay!
Um diddle diddle diddle, um diddle ay!
Um diddle diddle diddle, um diddle ay!
Um diddle diddle diddle, um diddle ay!

So when the cat has got your tongue,
There's no need for dismay.
Just summon up this word and then you've got a lot to say.
But better use it carefully or it can change your life.
One night I said it to me girl and now me girl's me wife.

She's Su-per-cal-i-frag-il-is-tic-ex-pi-al-i-do-cious.
Even though the sound of it is something quite a-tro-cious,
If you say it loud enough, you'll always sound pre-co-cious!
Su-per-cal-i-frag-il-is-tic-ex-pi-al-i-do-cious!
Su-per-cal-i-frag-il-is-tic-ex-pi-al-i-do-cious!

'K' - The Friend of the Palate

The **soft palate** affects the way the voice resonates, vibrates, and the richness of the sound of our voices. It is essential that it remain flexible and strong for clear, distinct speaking and singing. If the **soft palate** has been weakened by Parkinson's, stroke, or simply aging, exercises that use **plosive** consonants **k** or hard **c** can be beneficial. Professional singers also use these types of exercises to help produce focus and resonance[13] in the voice.

The **palate** has two specific areas inside the mouth: 1) the boney **hard palate** lies directly behind the upper teeth and does not move or flex. 2) the **soft palate**, consisting of muscle and fibers sheathed in mucous membrane, is flexible and lies behind the **hard palate**. The entire **palate** area is sometimes referred to as the "roof of the mouth."

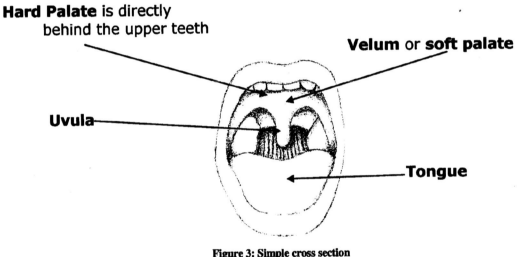

Hard Palate is directly behind the upper teeth

Velum or **soft palate**

Uvula

Tongue

Figure 3: Simple cross section
of human mouth/oral cavity.

In normal speech and song the **soft palate** closes off the nasal cavity except when speaking **n**, **m**, and **ng,** which sounds like humming and allows a small amount of air to flow through the nose. Other than these exceptions, the **soft palate** closes when speaking. If it does not close completely, air will leak through the nasal cavity. The result is a distorted, nasalized sound, as if the person is "speaking through their nose." Exercises that improve movement and efficiency of the **soft palate** are beneficial.

---

[13] *American Heritage Dictionary.* Resonance: The intensification or prolongation of sound, especially of musical tone, produced by sympathetic vibration.

K: Vocalises (For Vocal Ease CD (gold) track # 9.)

Consonants **k** and **hard c** are designed to improve movement and efficiency of the **soft palate**.

1.
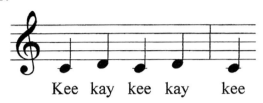

Kee kay kee kay   kee

2.
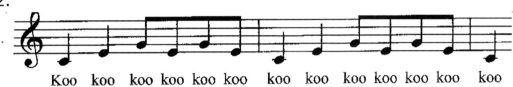

Koo koo koo koo koo koo   koo koo   koo koo koo koo   koo

3.
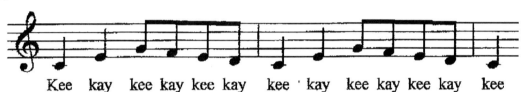

Kee kay kee kay kee kay   kee   kay   kee kay kee kay   kee

4.
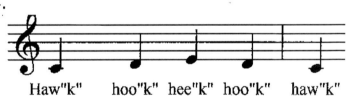

Haw"k"   hoo"k"   hee"k"   hoo"k"   haw"k"

5.
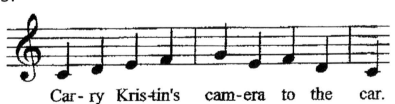

Car- ry Kris-tin's   cam-era to the   car.

6.
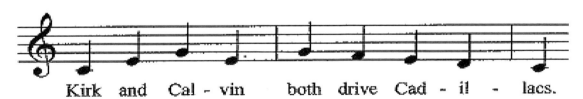

Kirk   and   Cal - vin   both   drive   Cad - il - lacs.

Time to Listen and Practice K

Sing-A-Long CD (blue) track #8.

Listen to this popular song from the 1950s — "Music! Music! Music!"

Each time you hear the words **music** and **nickelodeon** make the sound of the letter **K**. This is a great exercise for the soft palate.

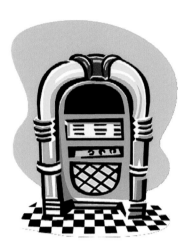

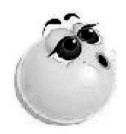

How many words can you think of that begin with **K** or hard **C**. Make a list and practice saying them a few times each day. Your soft palate will be very happy!

_____

_____

_____

_____

_____

Approximant Consonants: Adding Vitality

Approximant consonants are unique; their pronunciation is halfway between a vowel and a typical consonant. As is true throughout all speech, the relationship of vowels and consonants is ongoing; one influences the other. **Approximant consonants** require the use of tongue, lips, jaw and/or facial muscles, all of which are called **articulators**. The use of **articulators** is transforming to speech and song, adding clarity to words and vitality to our faces.

Approximant consonants W, Y, L, and sometimes R

W, and sometimes **Y** require the lips to come forward (like a kiss!).

L requires movement of the tongue, touching just behind the top front teeth.

R involves the use of the tongue and sometimes lips, when in conjunction with certain vowels.

Approximant Consonant Vocalises

Vocalises for Vocal Ease CD (gold) track # 10.

Keep facial muscles, lips, and tongue vitally engaged. Notice the subtle changes in your mouth, tongue, jaw, and face (articulators) created by each different vowel that follows the **approximant consonants**.

1. **R**   Robert Redford rarely rode the railroad.

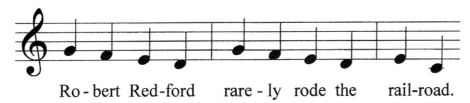

Ro - bert Red-ford   rare - ly rode the   rail-road.

2. **W**   Wally Williams wanted a white wagon.

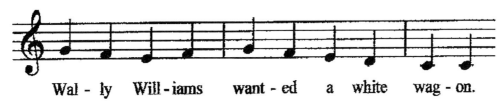

Wal - ly Will - iams   want - ed   a   white   wag - on.

3. **Y** Your youthful ways will work for you.

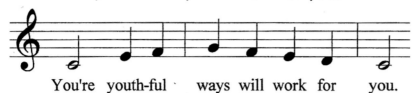

You're youth-ful · ways will work for you.

4. **L** Lacy lilies lined the lovely lane.

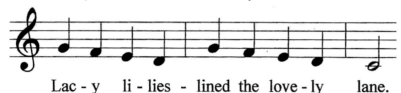

Lac - y li - lies - lined the love - ly lane.

Time to Sing-A-Long

***Sing-A-Long CD* (blue) track #9.**

Irving Berlin's 1954 hit "There's No Business, Like Show Business," is full of verve. It is hard to be lazy lipped as you sing this one!

"There's No Business Like Show Business"

There's no bus'ness like show bus'ness
Like no bus'ness I know
Ev'rything about it is appealing
Ev'rything the traffic will allow
Nowhere could you get that happy feeling
When you are stealing that extra bow

There's no people like show people
They smile when they are low
Even with a turkey that you know will fold
You may be stranded out in the cold
Still you wouldn't change it for a sack of gold

Let's go on with the show!
Let's go on with the show!

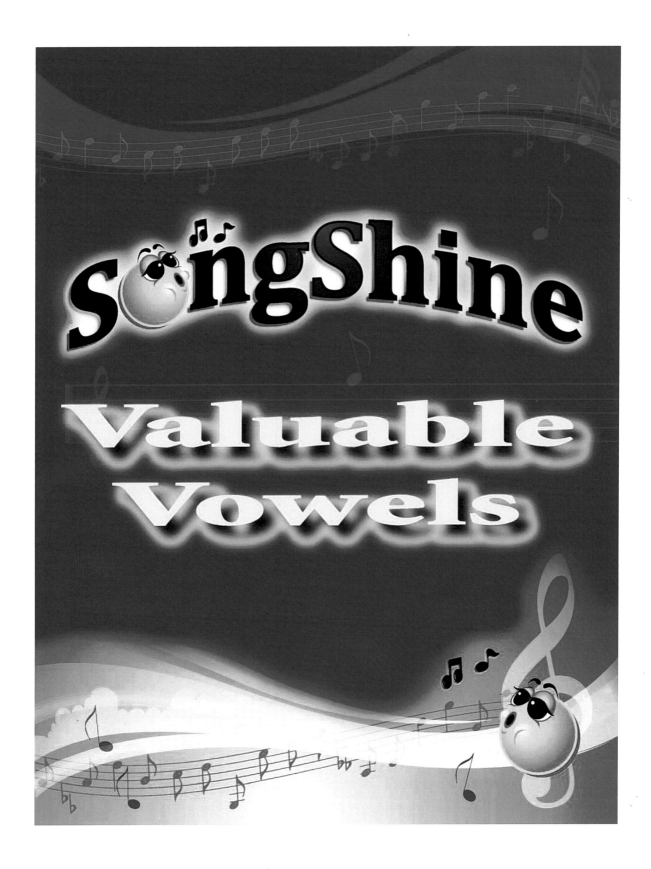

V. Valuable Vowels

If **consonants** are like springboards, **vowels** are like sailboats gliding over the lake. Moving air (breath) fills the sail (lungs) and sends the boat (vowel/word) skimming over the water (tone). Energy (air filled lungs) released from the **power pack** enables the vocal folds to vibrate normally, resulting in healthy tone.

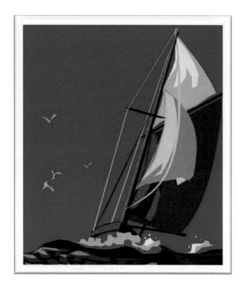

Air fills the sails and the boat glides across the water.

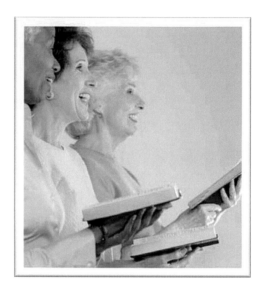

Air fills the lungs and is released through the vocal cords to produce singing tone.

Why Vowels are Valuable

Vowels are valuable not only because they create beautiful tone but because they give meaning to the words we speak or sing. Vowels carry expression, creating color, mood, and emotion. Language without vowels would sound like nothing more than a series of grunts, pops, gurgles, and miniature explosions of air released from within.

The English language has only 5 **vowels** (**A E I O U**), but many different sounds are created from them. As vowels combine, or are influenced by consonants, a variety of shadings occur. Understanding these sounds helps us train more effectively as **vocal athletes.** Ultimately, we are better able to maintain healthy, strong speaking and singing voices.

Pure Vowel Sounds

The most beautiful singing tone is created with **pure vowel sounds**. The **pure vowel sounds** of the Italian language explain why Italy has produced fabulous singers throughout the ages. English also has several **pure vowel sounds**.

Beautiful **pure vowel sounds** occur when there is only **one vowel sound** within a syllable. All of the words below have only **one vowel** and create **vowel sounds** that are **pure.** Speak each word below. Elongate (hold) the **vowel** and listen to the **pure single vowel sound**.

TAP   PET   SIT   ROB   COT   CUT

Using a comfortable note in the middle of your vocal range, sing the words you just spoke. Whether speaking or singing these examples there is only **one vowel sound**. Reminder: Use **noble posture** and engage your **power pack**. Sing:

TAP   PET   SIT   ROB   COT   CUT

In the examples below **two vowels** occur but only **one vowel sound** is heard. In these examples the **vowel sound** is still **pure.** Speak each word and listen to the **pure vowel sound**.

PAUSE   FRIEND   GREET   COOK   BEAST

Sing the same words on a comfortable pitch in your vocal range. This time notice three things: 1) the energy created by the **consonant** at the beginning of each word; this propels energy into the **vowel**;   2) the clarity of the **pure vowel**; 3) final consonants like **t** and **k** create a crisp ending.

PAUSE   FRIEND   GREET   COOK   BEAST

Pure Vowel Vocalises

Vocalises for Vocal Ease CD (gold) track # 11

Pure vowels sounds are "valuable" because they help develop beautiful singing tone.

1.

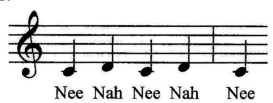

Nee Nah Nee Nah   Nee

2.

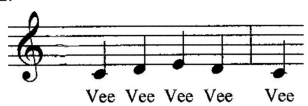

Vee Vee Vee Vee   Vee

3.

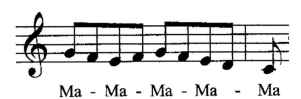

Ma - Ma - Ma - Ma - Ma

4.

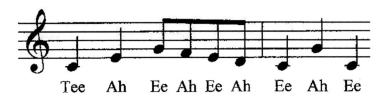

Tee Ah Ee Ah Ee Ah   Ee Ah Ee

5.

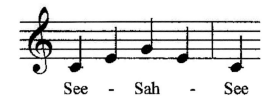

See - Sah - See

Time to Sing-A-Long

Sing-A-Long CD (blue) track # 10.

An excellent example of a song with **pure vowel sounds** and **consonants** that **energize,** is "Ja Da, Ja Da." This jaunty tune has moderate swingy rhythms and a nonsensical text. It was extremely popular from the early 1900's to the late 1940's.

"Ja Da"

Ja Da, Ja Da,
Ja Da, Ja Da, Jing, Jing, Jing,

Ja Da, Ja Da,
Ja Da, Ja Da, Jing, Jing, Jing,

That's a funny little bit of melody.
It's so soothing and appealing to me,
It goes Ja Da, Ja Da
Ja Da, Ja Da, Jing, Jing, Jing,

Ja Da, Ja Da,
Ja Da, Ja Da, Jing, Jing,
Ja Da, Ja Da, Jing, Jing,
Ja Da, Ja Da, Jing, Jing, Jing,

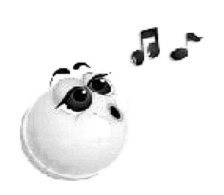

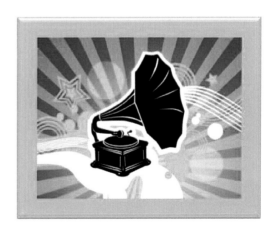

Vowel Placement

As you sing or speak, the naturally occurring **placement** or **position** of a vowel in your mouth influences the way you sound. Although there are a variety of subtle vowel positions, we will only examine the characteristics of three: **front, middle** and **back**. For example: Slowly speak the words below. Can you feel a difference in **placement** or **position** of each word?

KEEP	**CUP**	**COPE**
(front)	(middle)	(back)

Front vowels produce a bright forward tone, such as pure **E** in "keep".

Speak the following words which have **front vowels.** Where do you feel them? Are they forward? Can you sense them in the front part of your mouth?

FRONT VOWELS

E	in STEEP
I	in SIT
A	in TAPE
E	in PET
A	in PAT

Middle vowels, like **U** in "cup," are produced in the center of the mouth, but if not given adequate air flow or support from the **power pack,** can become throaty sounding. Speak the following words which are naturally placed in the **middle** of your mouth.

MIDDLE VOWELS

A	in <u>A</u>BOUT
U	in BUT
O	in COME

Back vowels, like **O** in "hold," are produced in the back of the mouth and can easily become dark and throaty without adequate airflow.

BACK VOWELS

OO	**in HOOT**
OO	**in BOOK**
O	**in BOAT**
AU	**in CAUSE**
O	**in COLD**

Understanding where vowel sounds are placed can help us communicate more effectively. All the things we are learning about **consonants** and **vowels** become **tools to keep us in the communication game longer**. Whether singing or speaking, understanding the optimum placement for vowels helps create beautiful tone. Like a gymnast with perfect placement on a balance beam, there is an ideal place for each **vowel sound**.

Using Your Brain to Trick and Train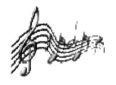

Sometimes practicing a simple trick can add clarity and beauty to singing or speaking. If **back** or **mid-vowels** sound throaty, try this trick: **Use a brighter/forward vowel to influence the darker/back vowel**. For example: Speak the word "cause." Sense the placement: **back/dark**. Now speak the word "keys," which is **bright/forward**. Practice alternately speaking the two words:

keys   cause   keys   cause   keys   cause

Another trick is to think the **brighter** vowel sound as you speak or sing the **darker** vowel. As your brain thinks the **brighter vowel**, it will influence the sound of the **darker** vowel, bringing it further forward. This type of exercise helps you maintain clear, bright, distinct speech and song.

Diphthongs

A **diphthong** (sometimes called a **shadow**) is a secondary **vowel sound** that is heard after the first or primary **vowel sound**. The English language presents an interesting challenge to singers and speakers because of **diphthongs.** Each word below has a **diphthong** or **shadow.** Speak the following words slowly and notice the influence of the secondary sound

COUCH   COW   BROIL   BOY   STATE   STOW

If equal emphasis is given to both the primary and secondary sound, the word becomes distorted.   Example: **COUCH** would sound like **CAH-OOCH**; **COW** would sound like **CAH-OO**, etc.   When a **diphthong** or **shadow** occurs **always emphasize the primary sound**.

The examples below are words that have secondary sounds or **diphthongs.** In these single syllable words the **primary vowel** sound is influenced by a **consonant(s)**. Speak slowly and listen to the vowel as it glides along, influenced by the consonant that follows.

GATE   BOY   CLOWN   SIGN   BABE

GRACE   BLAZE   PRICE   BITE   TAKE

Fine, well-trained athletes master "technique" in order to develop skill and beautiful form. Likewise, a fine singer with "excellent technique" can sing skillfully with beautiful tone by emphasizing the **primary vowel sound**. Let the **diphthongs fall away**.

Although **diphthongs** are common in the English language, the most beautiful singing tone is created when **pure vowels sounds are dominant**.

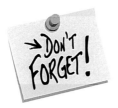

Diphthongs should   F
**   A**
**   L**
**   L   away**

Diphthongs: Let them Fall Away

Vocalises for Vocal Ease CD (gold) track # 12.

The exercises below contain a mixture of **pure vowel sounds** and **diphthongs**. Speak each word slowly. Circle the **diphthongs**.

1.

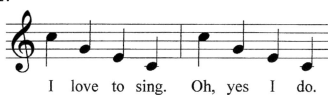

I love to sing. Oh, yes I do.

2.

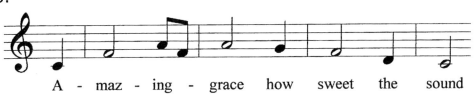

The sun is too bright.

3.

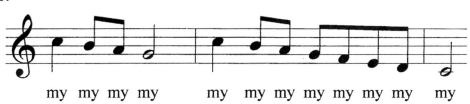

A - maz - ing - grace how sweet the sound

Answers: (1.) "I" "Oh"　(2.) "bright"　(3.) "amazing" "grace" "how" "sound"

Vocalises for Vocal Ease CD (gold) track # 13.

As you practice these vocalises, relax your jaw, sing on the **primary vowel sound** and **let diphthongs fall away**.

1.

my my my my　my my my my my my my　my

2.

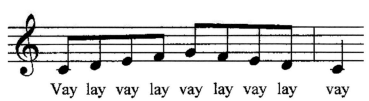

Vay lay vay lay vay lay vay lay   vay

3.

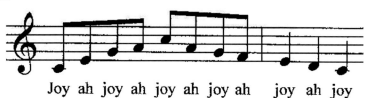

Joy ah joy ah joy ah joy ah   joy ah joy

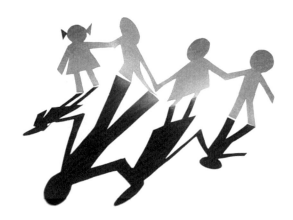

Diphthongs or shadows should fall away.

Below are words that contain **diphthongs.** Speak them and **allow** the **diphthong** to be prominent: sometimes hearing the negative helps reinforce the positive. Hearing the distortion will make you want to avoid the diphthong.

night   my   tight   our   shine   bright   light   might   may   they   now

Repeat the same words, but this time elongate the primary vowel and let the **diphthong fall away**.

night   my   tight   our   shine   bright   light   might   may   they   now

Time to Sing-A-Long

SongShine Sing-A-Long CD (blue) track #11.

The lyrics of this song, from Meredith Wilson's <u>The Music Man,</u> contain all the words you practiced speaking on the previous page. For the most beautiful tone, always allow the **diphthongs** or **shadows** to **fall away**.

"Goodnight, My Someone"

Goodnight, my someone, goodnight, my love,

Sleep tight, my someone, sleep tight, my love,

Our star is shining its brightest light

For goodnight, my love for goodnight.

Sweet dreams be yours, dear, if dreams there be;

Sweet dreams to carry you close to me,

I wish they may and I wish they might.

Now goodnight, my someone, goodnight.

Goodnight, goodnight, goodnight.

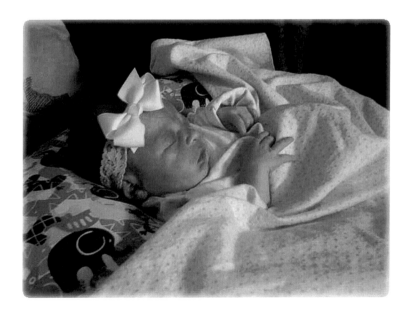

"Sweet dreams be yours, dear..."

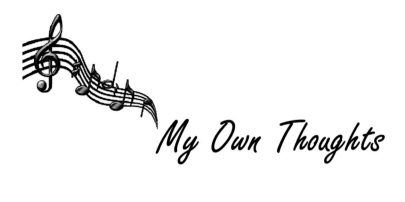

My Own Thoughts

What Really Makes Me Happy?

_____

_____

_____

_____

_____

What Puts a Song in My Heart?

_____

_____

_____

_____

_____

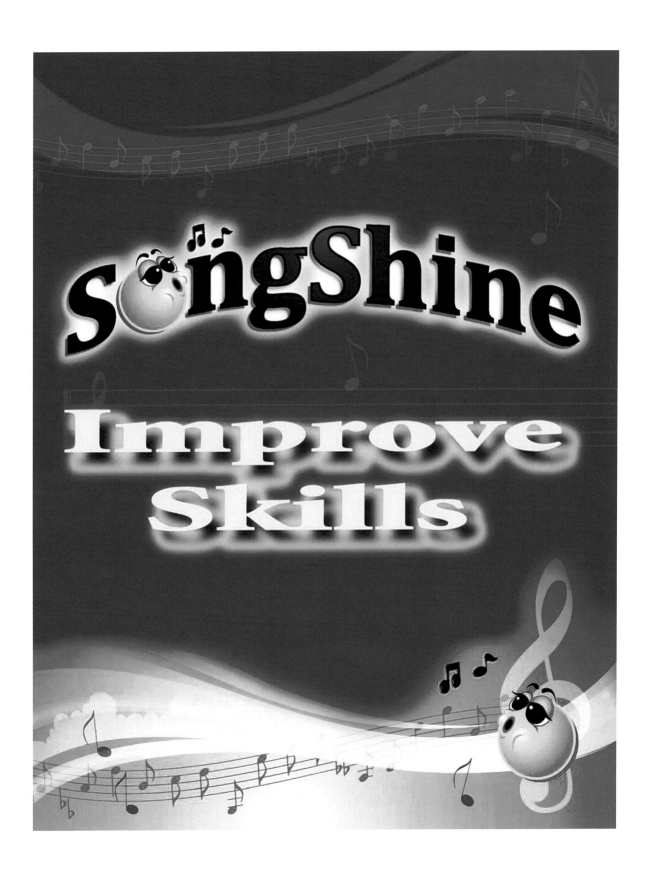

VI. Improving Your Skill

Stopping Tone: A Stealth Operation

Stopping **tone** is easy when there is a **consonant** at the end of a word; the consonant does the work for you automatically and cleanly. When a **vowel** is at the end of a word, the breath must continue to flow until the tone stops. The easiest way to learn to stop tone cleanly is to **take in a small amount of air, gently and silently, at the exact moment you want to stop the tone.** It is like a **"stealth operation:"** no one knows you are doing it, but the results are always perfect! The tone stops exactly where you want it to.

As you sing the exercise below, notice how the middle abdominals engage as you take a **gentle silent breath**; the tone stops immediately and cleanly.

Beginning and ending a **tone** requires two elements: brain and breath.

Use a gentle silent breath (stealth operation) at the end of each word.

Vocalises for Vocal Ease CD (gold) track #14.

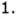1.

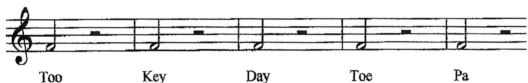

| Too | Key | Day | Toe | Pa |

The **gentle silent breath** technique puts you in control of your singing voice. It is also an invaluable technique for group or choral singing because it allows the group to follow the conductor's direction and stop the tone with absolute precision. Remember: brain and breath allow you to become a skilled **vocal athlete**. Stopping tone cleanly is like a football player catching or stopping the ball at exactly the "right" moment.

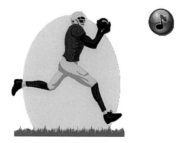
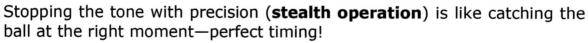

Stopping the tone with precision (**stealth operation**) is like catching the ball at the right moment—perfect timing!

Starting Tone: H—Helping Avoid Glottal Fry

Starting tone on a **vowel** requires special care. Because **H** automatically engages the **power pack**, it "helps" the speaker or singer prevent a raspy sound known as **glottal fry** or **scraping of the glottis**. This usually occurs because of inadequate air flow when a word begins with a vowel. In simple terms, the vocal cords are **scraping** rather than **vibrating** in a healthy manner.

Mosby's Medical dictionary (8th ed. 2009) defines **glottal fry** as "the raspy or croaking ("froglike") quality of the voice in its lowest register. It results from loose closure of the glottis that allows air to bubble through, giving rise to a series of low-pitched pops and rattles." If your voice has **glottal fry** you are probably not engaging the **power pack.** To avoid "pops and rattles" consistent airflow is required when initiating and sustaining tone. People with constant **glottal fry** have more laryngitis and hoarseness because of wear and tear on the vocal cords

Voices affected by Parkinson's or speech challenges after a stroke, will find it important to use the **H** technique to insure a proper amount of airflow. Adequate airflow results in clearer diction and a healthier voice.

Speak the **vowel sounds** below and listen for **glottal fry.** If you hear gurgles, rasps, or pops, you have not released enough breath to allow the vocal cords to vibrate normally.

EE	**EH**	**AH**	**OH**	**OO**

This time try speaking the following words, all of which begin with a vowel.

Remember to **think H** as you speak each word.

ARM	**EAR**	**INK**	**OFF**	**UP**
APPLE	**ENGLISH**	**IMPULSE**	**OPAL**	**UNDER**

Now try speaking an entire sentence, full of words that begin with vowels.

Prepare with **noble posture**, engage your **power pack**, and **think H**. The old adage will prove true, "practice makes perfect."

Elizabeth and Edward are under an ancient elm enjoying an autumn evening.

Vocalises: Avoiding Glottal Fry

Vocalises for Vocal Ease (gold) track # 15.

Check for **noble posture**. Use your **power pack.** Take a breath after each arrow. ⇩ Listen for **glottal fry** when you start or stop the tone.

1.

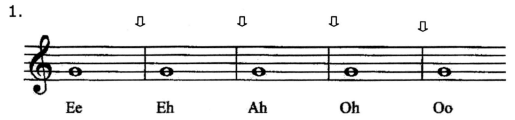

Use an **H** to start each tone. Notice the **absence of glottal fry**. Take a full breath before you sing each word. Remember to check your posture: Is it **noble**? Have you engaged your **power pack**? Breathe between words.

2.

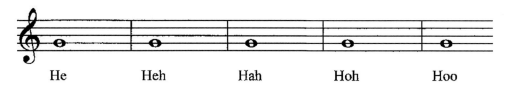

This time only **think H** preceding the vowel. Engage your **power pack**. Remember: **THINK H,** but do not actually sing it. Breathe between words.

3.

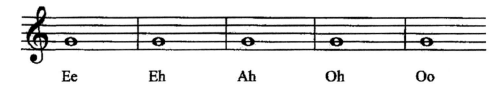

As you master these singing techniques, allow them to carry over into speech. The **absence of glottal fry means your breath supply is adequate** and you are gaining strength and control of your voice.

Listen to people speaking on the radio, TV. Do their voices flow freely or do you hear **glottal fry**? If you hear gurgles, pops and raspy sounds you are hearing **glottal fry.**

The next time your phone rings, before you say "hello," remember to take an **intentional breath**, fill your **power pack**, and let **H** be your **helper.** Your voice will be clearer, stronger, and vibrant **without glottal fry.**

Artistry and Control: Crescendo/Decrescendo/Legato

Singing with expression requires being able to change volume levels. When the music calls for the tone to gradually become louder you *crescendo* (pronounced creh-shen'-doh), which means become **gradually louder**. To accomplish this you must **increase air flow** from the **power pack**. The mid-abdominal muscles remain flexed and the chest wall should not collapse. To learn this technique, sing one note on **Nee**. Gradually increase the volume. The sign for *crescendo* is seen below. Remember to stop the tone by taking a **quick silent breath**.

Vocal Exercises for Crescendo, Decrescendo and Legato

Vocalises for Vocal Ease CD (gold) track # 16.

1. Crescendo

Nee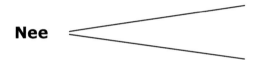

Decrescendo (pronounced deh'-creh-shen'-doh) means gradually softer.

The abdominal muscles remain engaged and the chest wall must not collapse. To stop the tone, use the **silent breath** technique. The musical sign for *decrescendo* is seen below.

2. Decrescendo

Nee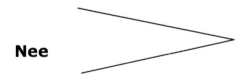

3. *Legato* (pronounced leh-gah'-toh means **smooth and flowing**.

Sing the exercise on one breath, flowing smoothly from one note to the next.

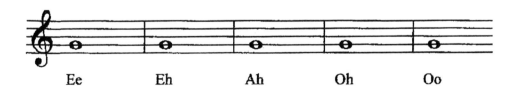

Ee   Eh   Ah   Oh   Oo

Time to Sing-A-Long

SongShine Sing-A-Long (blue) Track # 12.

"Oklahoma!" presents an excellent opportunity to practice several techniques: 1) avoiding glottal fry on words that begin or end with vowels, 2) singing plosive **K** sounds to improve mobility of the soft palate, 3) using *crescendo* to increase respiratory function.

"Oklahoma"

Oklahoma,
Where the wind comes sweepin' down the plain
And the wavin' wheat
Can sure smell sweet
When the wind comes right behind the rain.
Oklahoma!
Every night my honey lamb and I
Sit alone and talk
And watch a hawk
Makin' lazy circles in the sky.
We know we belong to the land,
And the land we belong to is grand.
And when we say:
Yee-ow! A-yip-i-o-ee-ay!
We're only sayin',
You're doin' fine, Oklahoma!
Oklahoma,
O-K-L-A-H-O-M-A, Oklahoma!   **Yee-ow!**

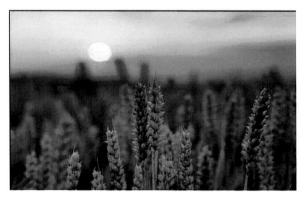

"and the wavin' wheat

can sure smell sweet..."

Sing-A-Long CD (blue) track # 13.

"Edelweiss," from Rodgers and Hammerstein's famous and much loved musical, _The Sound of Music_, requires 1) smooth flowing **legato** tone (engage your **power pack**) and 2) avoiding **diphthongs** (sing on the primary vowel).

"Edelweiss"

Edelweiss,
Edelweiss,
Every morning you greet me.
Small and white,
Clean and bright,
You look happy to meet me.
Blossom of snow,
May you bloom and grow,
Bloom and grow forever –
Edelweiss,
Edelweiss,
Bless my homeland forever.

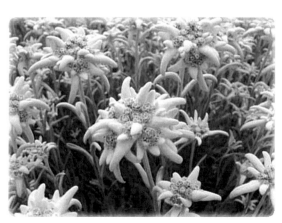

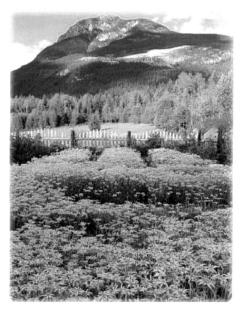

Edelweiss photos courtesy Mr. Peter Risch,
Golden, British Columbia

"…bless my homeland, forever."

Thankfulness

Today I am thankful for

_____

_____date _____

Today I am thankful for

_____

_____date _____

Today I am thankful for

_____

_____date _____

Today I am thankful for

_____

_____date _____

Today I am thankful for

_____

_____date _____

Today I am thankful for

_____

_____date _____

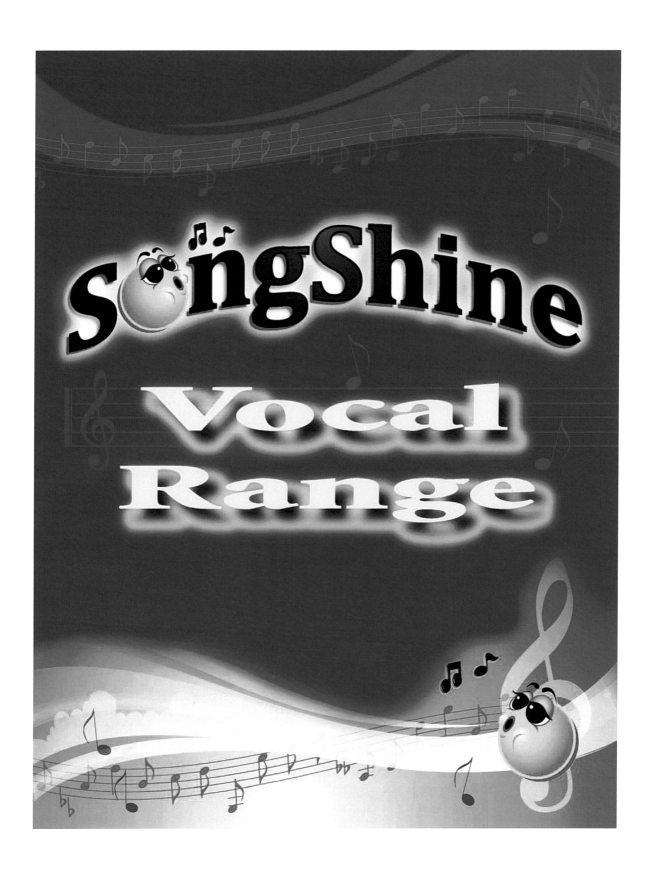

VII. Range Extension

A common voice characteristic of those with Parkinson's or stroke is flattened, monotone speech. Likewise, a common complaint of singers with aging voices is, "I have lost my high/low notes." In both cases **range** and **pitch** variation for speaking or singing has been diminished.

Vocal **range** includes all the pitches that can be sung without strain, from highest to lowest. Exercises that help increase **range** are beneficial to those who experience decreased **range** function. Limited **range,** however, is not exclusive to those with Parkinson's, stroke or aging voices. Even young singers frequently have limited **range**, usually due to poor vocal technique or fear.

Excellent vocal technique is the key to increasing **range** and eliminating fear when singing. Excellent vocal technique includes: 1) **noble posture**, 2) fully engaged **power pack**, 3) relaxed jaw, 4) relaxed soft palate.

Upward Range Extension: The Yawn

A simple technique for accessing upper notes in the vocal range is the "yawn-sigh" technique. Open your mouth as if you are yawning and very relaxed. Breathe in through the mouth and allow the soft palate to rise. A relaxed, raised soft palate is the key to extending the range upward. Simply practice yawning!

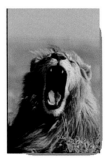

Vocalises for Vocal Ease CD (gold) track # 17.

The exercise below uses **H** to engage the **power pack** and abdominals. Most important: **Think yawn for upward range extension**.

1.

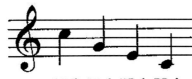

Hai Yai Yai Yai

Notice the helpful elements in the exercise above.

    a. It begins with 'H', which is a "helper" generating breath flow.

    b. 'H' is followed by a, which creates an "**ah**" sound. This allows the **soft palate** to relax and rise and the jaw to open like a yawn.

    c. The final **sound** of each word is a slight **E sound**, which is **bright forward**. This keeps the sound from going back into your throat.

The entire exercise is an example of tricking your voice with your brain.

The exercise below also requires the feeling of **yawn**; open space with raised soft palate. The word "Oh" helps establish the feeling of openness. You may also substitute "Ah" for "Oh." Always think of **yawning**.

2.

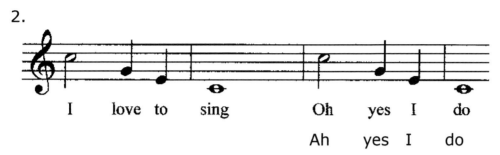

Notice two things in the exercise below:

a. **Sk** in the word "sky" creates a springboard effect, propelling energy into the **vowel sound**.

b. The word "sky" has a **shadow** or **diphthong**. Sing on the **primary vowel sound** and let the **diphthong** fall away as seen in the second line.

3.

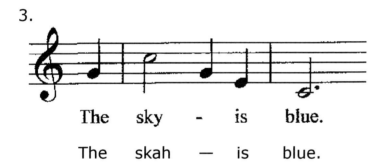

4.

Keep the abdominals flexed and an open and relax the jaw on "Ah."

Think of **yawning** on the highest note. Try adding **s** before 'ah' for extra energy on the highest note. Add an **s** to 'ah' to increase energy.

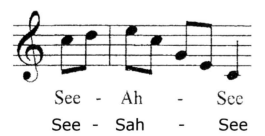

Think of yawning on "Ah." Also practice adding **S** in front of "Ah." This will increase energy on the highest note: See Sah See.

5.

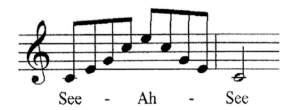

See - Ah - See

Downward Range Extension: Buzzzzzzzzzz!

Z creates energy. Say the word "buzz," making a continuous "BUZZZZZ"

Vocalises for Vocal Ease CD (gold) track # 18.

Sing an energetic **Z** with one "Zah" and then sing "Zah" on every note.

1.

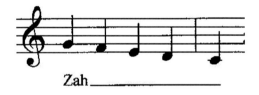

Zah_____

Zah zah zah zah zah

Relax the jaw. Keep abdominals flexed.

2.

Mah mah mah mah mah

Energize each **Z** and relax the jaw.

3.

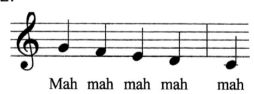

Zee Zah Zee Zah

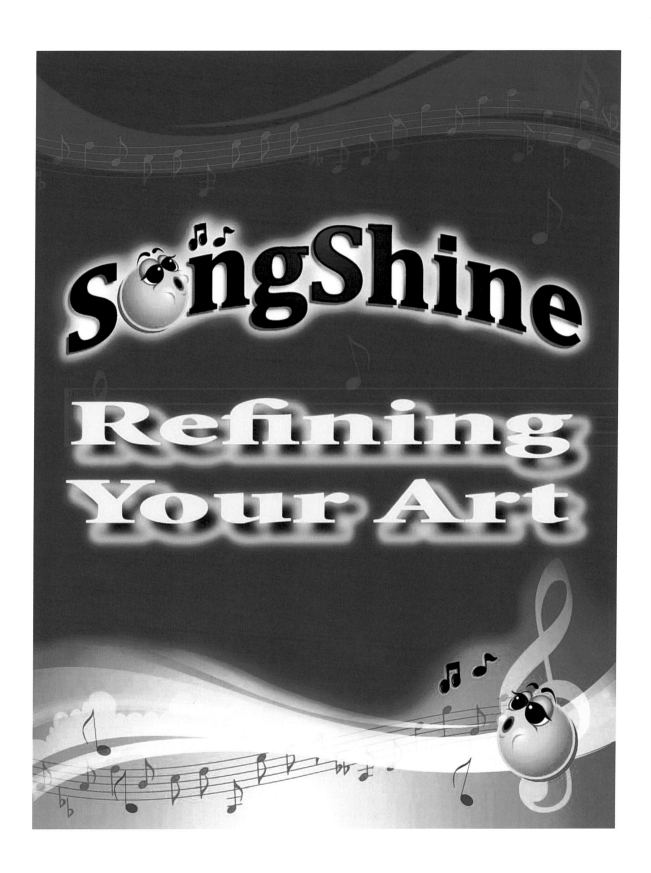

VIII. Refining Your Art

Legato—Smooth Flowing Tone

Beautiful speaking and singing occurs when words or tone flow evenly. With aging, Parkinson's, or stroke, the voice becomes uneven, with breaks and stops and starts. Think of an Olympic figure skater moving smoothly and beautifully over the ice; likewise the singer's voice, when singing *legato,* should flow smoothly from one word to the next. You will need adequate breath supplied by engaging your **power pack**. Remember, your posture and the Olympic skater's posture should always remain **noble**.

Vocalises for Vocal Ease CD (gold) track # 19.

Legato **vocalises**—keep the breath flowing from one **m** to the next **m**.

1.

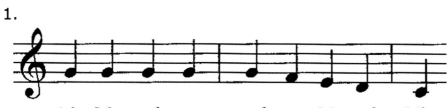

Relaxed jaw and flowing breath from one **M** to the next.

2.

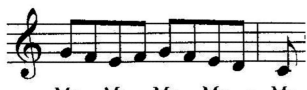

Keep a continuous flow of breath and relaxed jaw.

3.

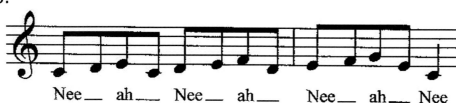

"Th" energizes the vowels in the words below. Sing smooth flowing *legato* in the second measure.

4.

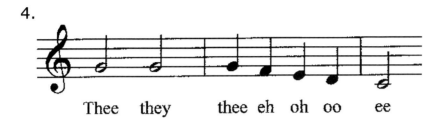

Thee they thee eh oh oo ee

Think of gliding down a musical staircase.

5.

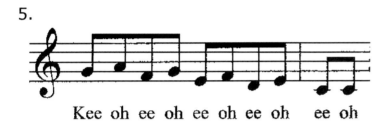

Kee oh ee oh ee oh ee oh ee oh

Fill the **power pack** and keep the breath flowing continuously.

6.

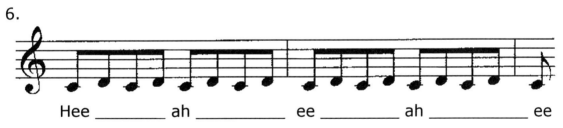

Hee _____ ah _____ ee _____ ah _____ ee

Each word should flow evenly into the next word, but be clearly understood.

7.

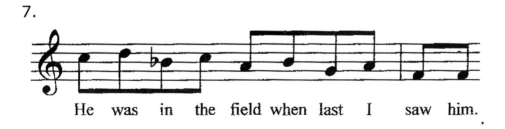

He was in the field when last I saw him.

Adding Agility Requires Precision and Flexibility

Songs that require vocal **agility** need to move with **flexibility** and **precision**. Gaining vocal **flexibility** and **agility** is like learning to figure skate. A figure skater practices "figures" each day, slowly and with precision. Only after the figures are mastered can skaters attempt the beautiful leaps, spins, and quick turns demanded of them.

Likewise, **agility** and **flexibility** exercises require a routine.

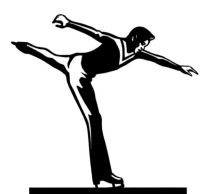

1. Employ your acquired skills concerning posture and breathing.

2. Vocalize with your regular vocal exercises.

3. Become familiar with the **flexibility** and **agility** exercises presented in this chapter.

4. Sing with the Vocalises for Vocal Ease CD or the Five Day Vocal Workout CD.

5. Practice each new **flexibility** and **agility** exercise slowly.

6. Gradually increase speed as you become comfortable with each exercise.

In addition to improving agility, they also add strength and can help continue to increase vocal range.

Vocalises for Vocal Ease CD (gold) track # 20.

Agility and Strength Vocalises. Take a breath where indicated by the arrows.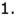

1.

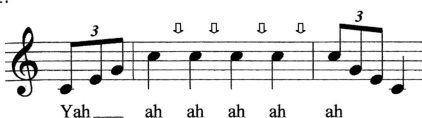

Yah____ ah ah ah ah ah

Think short bursts of energy/breath on each note. Do not try to take a breath between each note. Pretend your are Santa Claus singing "Hoh-hoh-hoh-hoh-hoh!" and "Hee-hee-hee-hee-hee."

2.

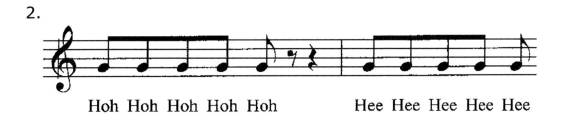

Hoh Hoh Hoh Hoh Hoh   Hee Hee Hee Hee Hee

Take a full breath; sing the word "Tee" softly, then **crescendo** (get louder) as you sing "ah." Use only one breath for the entire exercise.

3.

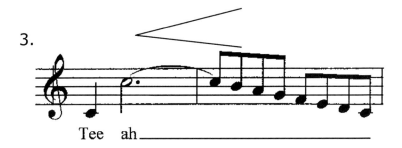

Tee ah

Adding flexibility and agility exercises to your routine can increase your singing skills. Like an ice skater moving with flexibility and speed over the ice, you can improve your ability by simply incorporating this routine into your daily vocal regimen as a vocal athlete.

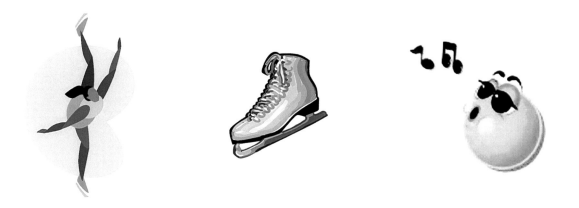

Time to Sing-A-Long

Sing-A-Long CD (blue) track #14.

Here's the perfect test for your new skills: As a vocal athlete you will no doubt be able to climb this mountain with ease. Wear **noble posture**, fill your **power pack**, and plant your boots firmly on the trail. When you reach the top, let me be the first to say, **"CONGRATULATIONS, YOU MADE IT TO THE SUMMIT!"**

"Climb Ev'ry Mountain"

Climb ev'ry mountain,
Search high and low,
Follow ev'ry byway,
Every path you know.
Climb ev'ry mountain,
Ford ev'ry stream,
Follow ev'ry rainbow
Till you find your dream.
A dream that will need
all the love you can give
Ev'ry day of your life
for as long as you live.
Climb ev'ry mountain,
Ford ev'ry stream,
Follow ev'ry rainbow
Till you find your dream.

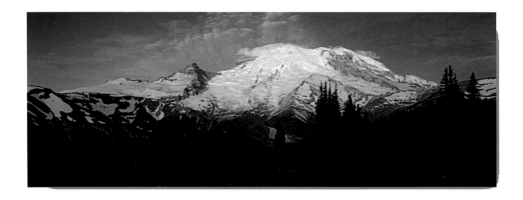

Mt. Rainier Photo used by permission - Lee Mann Photography.

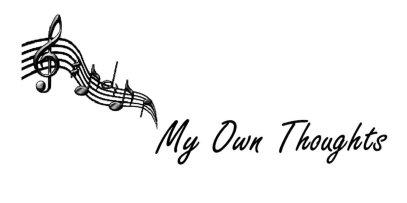

My Own Thoughts

What are my favorite sports?   Why?

_____

_____

_____

What are my favorite songs   Why?

_____

_____

_____

Do sports and music have anything in common?   What?

_____

_____

_____

What could I do today to make someone happy?

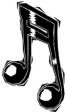

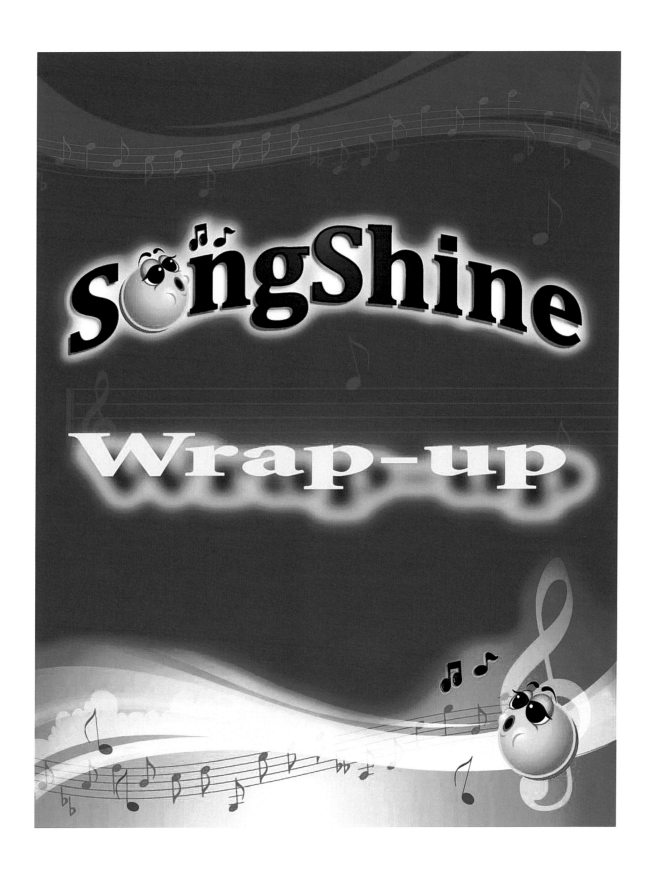

SongShine

Wrap-up

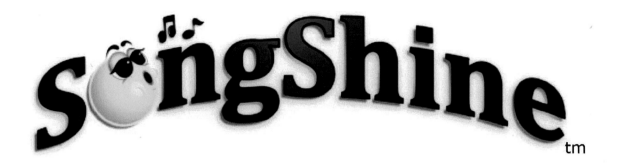

IX. The Wrap Up

Stay In the Game

Having nearly completed your *SongShine* textbook, and having been engaged in daily vocal workouts, your voice should have gained clarity, strength, and agility. Your speaking voice should also be stronger and clearer.

It is my hope that your experience in *SongShine* has been positive, that you have come to appreciate the wonderful "built-in" instrument each human being has been given—a voice. Always think of your voice as a special gift. Every voice is unique; every voice can become more pleasing. Give your voice the best possible care by committing to a regular regimen of vocal exercise.

As the saying goes, "The ball is in your court." What will you do with it? There is no need to sit on the sidelines. I am going to believe you will continue to play the communication game for as long as you live. You have the skill—play it well.

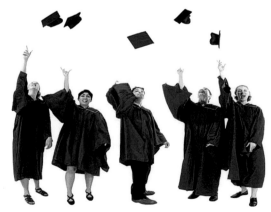

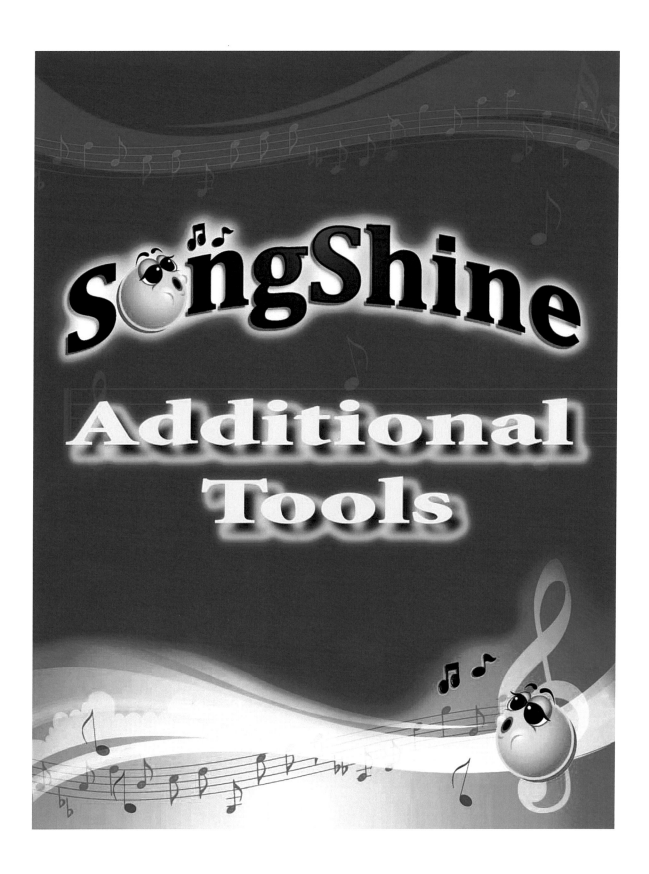

X. Additional Tools

Going to the Vocal Gym SongShine Style

Five-Day Vocal Workout

The **SongShine Five-Day Vocal Workout** provides five sets of vocal exercises to be practiced, one set each day. It's like going to the gym for vocal athletes. Instead of treadmills, rowing machines, stair masters, and weights, you will work out with humming, diction exercises, breath support, soft palate strengtheners, smooth flowing tone production, range extension, and vocal strength building. Each exercise is designed to keep your voice limber and healthy. As you play the **SongShine Five-Day Vocal Workout CD (white),** listen to the spoken instructions and sing along. Although written music is provided for you, it is not necessary to read music to sing the vocalises. When you are familiar with all the exercises, you may want to repeat one or two of the days in order to have a 6 or 7 day routine. Most important: **enjoy** your vocal workout.

Tips for an effective vocal workout

1. Choose a quiet place to practice.

2. Choose a regular time and establish a habit.

3. Whether sitting or standing, use **noble posture**.

4. Breathe deeply. Fill your **power pack** with oxygen/air.

5. The vocalises included in the **Five Day Vocal Workout CD** cover the topics included in your **SongShine** text book. Use your textbook to refresh your memory.

6. Your best friend is a mirror: Observe posture, facial expression and a relaxed jaw.

7. Remember: Practice makes perfect. But most important—**ENJOY!**

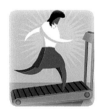 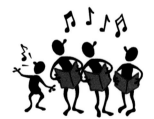 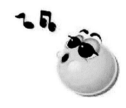

Become a vocal athlete!

Be A Winner
Use Your Five-Day Vocal Workout CD

Each time you sing-a-long with your Five-Day Vocal Workout CD it is like doing vocal calisthenics; you are exercising your voice. If you never exercise your physical muscles they will grow weak; the same is true with your voice. As you vocalize properly you also strengthen and help maintain a stronger speaking voice. Of all the games we play in life, the communication game may be the most important. Staying vocally fit will keep you in the communication game longer; you, your friends and your family will all be winners: that's a win-win!

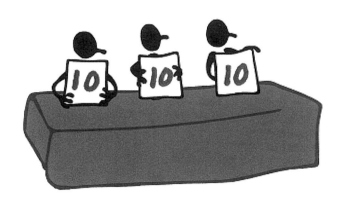

And the WINNER IS: _____

(Your name goes here)

Track #	**Day #**	**Printed Music**
Track 1	Day 1	page 106
Track 2	Day 2	page 108
Track 3	Day 3	page 110
Track 4	Day 4	page 112
Track 5	Day 5	page 114

Day 1
Five-Day Vocal Workout

1. Humming

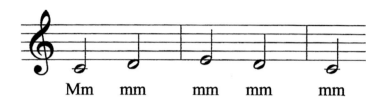

2. Diction and Relaxed Jaw

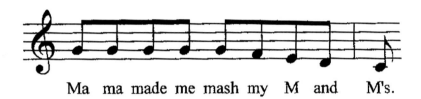

3. Soft Palate Flexibility. Rounded Lips.

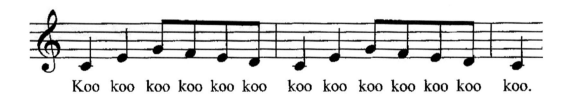

4. Resonance and Brightness

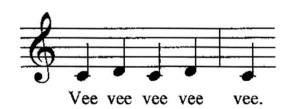

5. Relaxed Jaw and Upward Range Extension

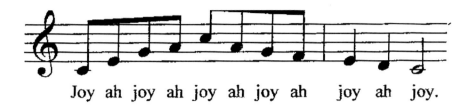

Joy ah joy ah joy ah joy ah   joy ah joy.

6. Range Extension Upward with Yawn/Sigh

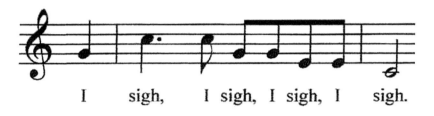

I   sigh,   I sigh, I sigh, I   sigh.

7. Range Extension Downward, Vibrant 'Z' and Dropped Jaw

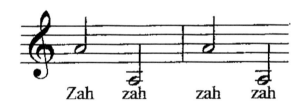

Zah   zah   zah   zah

8. Smooth Flowing Tone and Flexible Lips

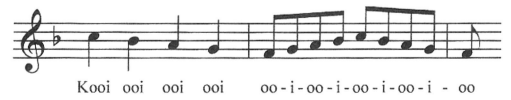

Kooi ooi ooi ooi   oo-i-oo-i-oo-i-oo-i - oo

Day 2
Five-Day Vocal Workout

1. Humming

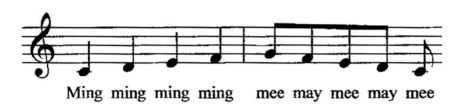

2. Resonance

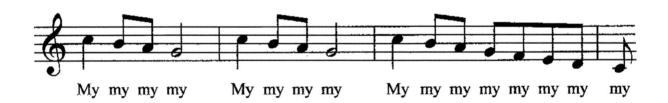

3. Relaxed Jaw

4. Soft Palate Flexibility

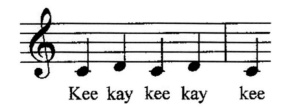

5. Range Extension Upward and Yawn/Sigh

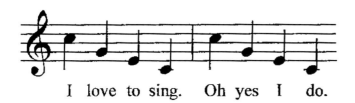

I love to sing. Oh yes I do.

6. Upward Range Extension and Flexibility

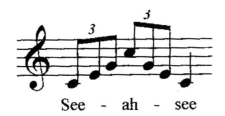

See - ah - see

7. Resonance and Flowing Tone

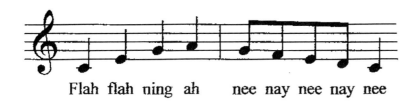

Flah flah ning ah   nee nay nee nay nee

8. Smooth Flowing Tone

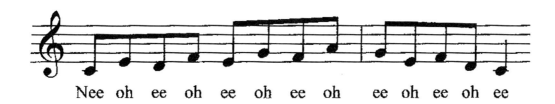

Nee oh ee oh ee oh ee oh   ee oh ee oh ee

Day 3
Five-Day Vocal Workout

1. Humming with Glissando. Glissando means to glide from one pitch to another.

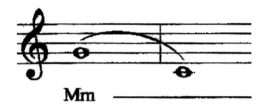

Mm ————

2. Resonance

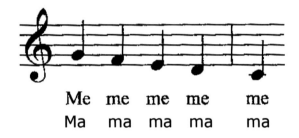

Me me me me   me
Ma ma ma ma   ma

3. Breath Flow and Relaxed Jaw

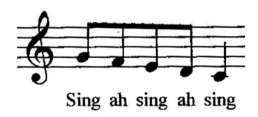

Sing ah sing ah sing

4. Soft Palate Flexibility

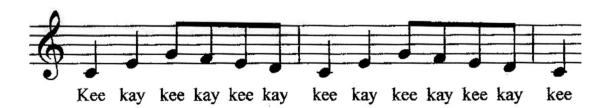

Kee kay kee kay kee kay   kee kay kee kay kee kay   kee

5. Range Extension Upward with Relaxed Jaw

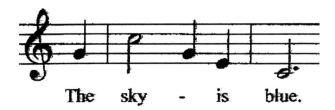

The sky - is blue.

6. Smooth Flowing Tone

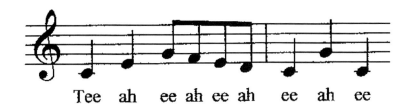

Tee ah ee ah ee ah ee ah ee

7. Diction and Plosive Consonants

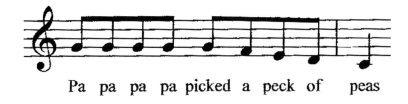

Pa pa pa pa picked a peck of peas

8. Smooth Flowing Tone and Fine Diction

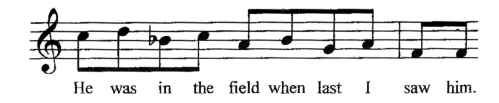

He was in the field when last I saw him.

Day 4
Five-Day Vocal Workout

1. Humming

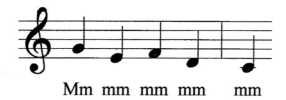

2. Resonance

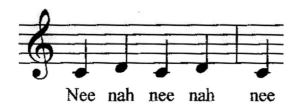

3. Resonance

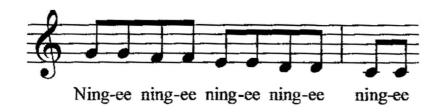

4. Tongue Movement and Diction

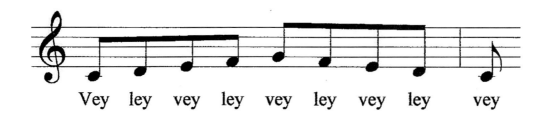

5. Soft Palate Flexibility

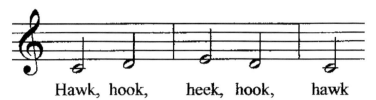

Hawk, hook, heek, hook, hawk

6. Smooth Flowing Tone

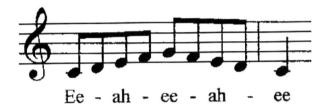

Ee - ah - ee - ah - ee

7. Range Extension Upward and Flowing Tone

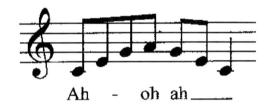

Ah - oh ah_____

8. Strength and Breath

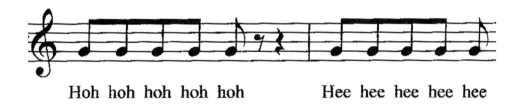

Hoh hoh hoh hoh hoh   Hee hee hee hee hee

9. Flexibility and Breath Flow

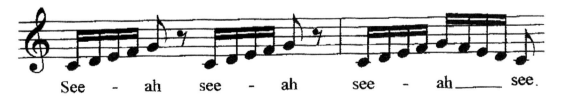

See - ah see - ah see - ah_____ see.

Day 5
Five-Day Vocal Workout

1. Humming

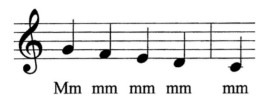

2. Resonance

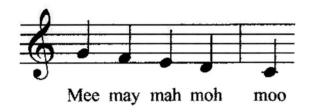

3. Resonance

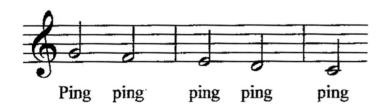

4. Soft Palate Flexibility

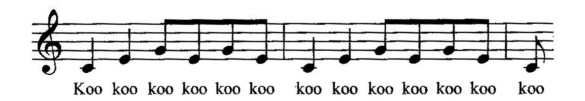

5. Diction and Breath

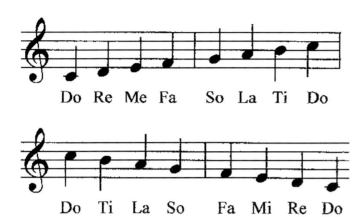

6. Breath and Diction

Sing all the words on one note. Repeat as you descend the scale.

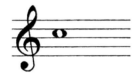

Do Re Mi Fa So La Ti Do

7. Upward Range Extension and Relaxed Jaw

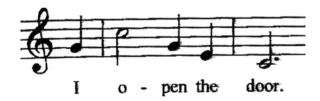

8. Diction

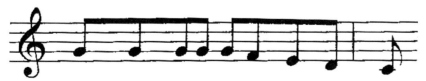

9. Strength Builder

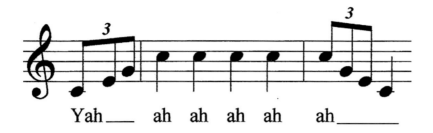

Yah __ ah ah ah ah ah _____

10. Smooth Flowing Tone

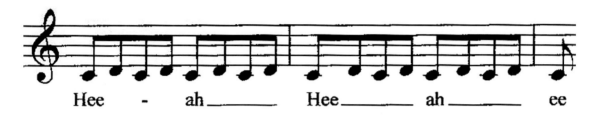

Hee - ah _____ Hee _____ ah _____ ee

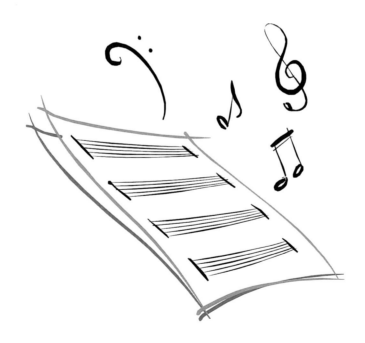

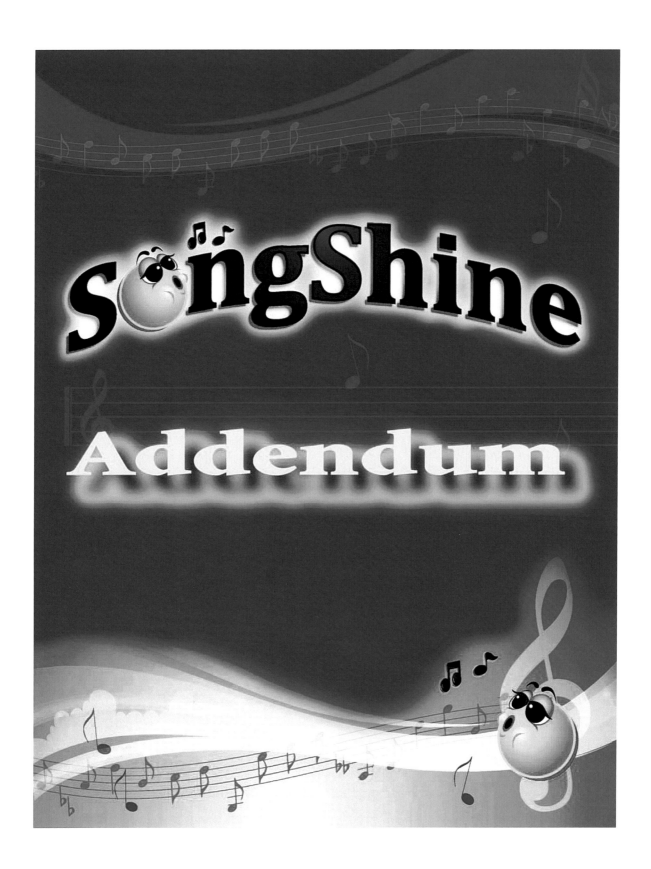

Appendix A
Vocalises for Vocal Ease CD (gold)
Page Location in Textbook

CD Track #	Subject	Textbook Page #
1	Introduction	38
2	**S**-ing for Energized **S**-ound	38
3	Singing Numbers (Breath)	39
4	Italian Scale (Breath)	40
5	Humming Exercises	52
6	Resonance and Humming: **N & M**	53
7	Plosive Consonant Energizers	58
8	Plosive and Fricative Vocalises	60
9	Soft Palate Flexibility: **K** and Hard **C**	65
10	Approximants: Adding Vitality	67
11	Pure Vowel Vocalises	72
12	Recognizing Diphthongs	77
13	Diphthongs Fall Away	77
14	Stopping Tone: A Stealth Operation	82
15	Starting Tone: **H** Avoiding Glottal Fry	84
16	Crescendo, Decrescendo, Legato	85
17	Range Extension Upward	90
18	Range Extension Downward	92
19	Smooth Flowing Tone (Legato)	94
20	Agility, Flexibility, and Strength	96

Appendix B
SongShine Sing-A-Long CD (blue)

CD Track #	Title	Textbook Page #
1	Do-Re-Mi	40
2	Wunderbar	42
3	Yankee Doodle	49
4	California, Here I Come	50
5	Chim Chim Cher-ee	54
6	Sh-Boom	62
7	Supercalifragilisticexpialidocious	63
8	Music! Music! Music! (Put Another Nickel In)	66
9	There's No Business Like Show Business	68
10	Ja Da, Ja Da, Jing, Jing, Jing	73
11	Goodnight, My Someone	79
12	Oklahoma	86
13	Edelweiss	87
14	Climb Ev'ry Mountain	98

Appendix C
Five-Day Vocal Workout CD (white)
Corresponding Printed Music

Track #	Day #	Printed Music
Track 1	Day 1	page 106
Track 2	Day 2	page 108
Track 3	Day 3	page 110
Track 4	Day 4	page 112
Track 5	Day 5	page 114

Permission Acknowledgments

Goodnight, My Someone
from Meredith Wilson's THE MUSIC MAN
by Meredith Wilson
Copyright © 1957 (Renewed) FRANK MUSIC CORP. and MEREDITH WILSON MUSIC
All Rights Reserved
Reprinted by permission of Hal Leonard Corporation

Wunderbar
from KISS ME, KATE All Rights Reserved Lyrics Permission in Process
Words and Music by Cole Porter
Copyright © 1948 by Cole Porter
Copyright Renewed,
Assigned to John F. Wharton, Trustee of the Cole Porter Musical and Literary Property
Trusts
Chappell and Co. owner of publication and allied rights throughout the world
International Copyright secured   All Rights Reserved
Reprinted by permission of Hal Leonard Corporation

Sh-Boom (Life Could Be A Dream)
Words and Music by James Keyes, Claude Feaster, Carl Feaster, Floyd McRae and James
Edwards
Copyright © 1954 by Unichappell Music Inc.
Copyright Renewed
International Copyright Secured   All Rights Reserved
Reprinted by permission of Hal Leonard Corporation

"California, Here I Come"
by Buddy De Sylva and Joseph Meyer © 1924
Alfred Publishing (33-1/3 %) All Rights Reserved Conditional Lyrics Permission in
Process
Memory Lane (33-1/3%) All Rights Reserved Conditional Lyrics Permission Granted
Songwriters Guild of America (33-1/3%) All Rights Reserved
Conditional Lyrics Permission Granted

Mechanical Licenses for Recording of Sing A-Long Accompaniment CD Granted by Harry
Fox Agency:Songfile for: "Climb Ev'ry Mountain," "Do-Re-Mi," "Edelweiss," "Oklahoma,"
"Goodnight, My Someone," "There's No Business Like Show Business," "Wunderbar,"
"Music! Music! Music! ," "Sh-Boom," "California, Here I Come."

"Yankee Doodle"
 Public Domain Traditional Revolutionary War Song

"Ja Da, Ja Da"
by Bob Carleton, 1918, Public Domain

ADDENDUM: Permissions

Photo Permissions

Page 13 and 14: *SongShine* students in class. Permission granted by *SongShine Students*

Page 16: Roy and Ruthanna in the Sierra's. Photo courtesy Doug Mc Nair

Page 56: Roy Metzgar, Diver, Photo Permission granted by Mr. Roy Metzgar

Page 87: Edelweiss. Permission granted by Mr. Peter Risch Edelweiss Golden, British Columbia. http://edelweissgrowers.com

Page: 99: Mount Rainier. Permission granted by Mr. Lee Mann. http://www.leemannphotography.com

Figures

Figure 36: Human torso (page 12) drawn by Roy Metzgar.

Figure 46: Simple cross section of human head (page 22) drawn by Roy Metzgar.

Figure 64: Simple cross section of human mouth/oral cavity (page 39) drawn by Ashley Sheldon.

Poems

SongShine Singing Stars by Janet Huff (page 8) © July 2010 Permission granted by Janet Huff. Janet is a part of the Eisenhower Medical Center Rancho Mirage, CA *SongShine* group. Janet is a degreed music teacher, writer, and editor.

I'll Try by Roy Metzgar (page 18) © August 2010 Permission granted by Roy Metzgar

My Life Is But A Weaving (page 125) Author unknown, Public Domain

Printed Music

"SongShine Singing Stars" by Janet Huff, © July 2010, Permission granted Janet Huff.   Arranged Dorothy Anderson © October 2010, Permission granted Dorothy Anderson.

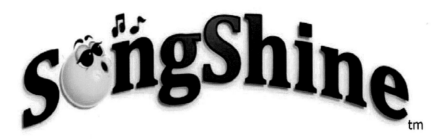

About The Author

Ruthanna has both bachelor's and master's degrees in music from the University of Michigan and a doctorate in music from the University of Washington. She has served on the faculty of four universities, Elderhostel, and been a guest lecturer for Grand Rounds and Continuing Education (Otolaryngology and Speech Pathology) at the University of Washington Medical School. Other lecture opportunities have included Virginia Mason Hospital, the University of Oregon, University of Victoria (British Columbia), Seattle Pacific University, and Shoreline Community College (WA).

She has presented solo concerts in the US, Canada, Switzerland, and over 200 concerts in Japan. While serving as director of the Phoenix Choir of Baltimore, she conducted concerts in France, Germany, Belgium and Netherlands. She was guest soloist on the "NBC Today Show" and has soloed with university and civic orchestras and choirs. During her tenure as musical director and conductor of the Harrisburg, PA Civic Opera, she made her orchestral conducting debut with Strauss's "Die Fledermaus." She has served as minister of music for several churches and has been a speaker for women's retreats and conferences.

Ruthanna teaches at Eisenhower Medical Center, Rancho Mirage, CA. In April 2010, she presented a lecture on *SongShine* at the 21st Annual International Arts in Healthcare Conference, Minneapolis, MN. She remains an active performer, singing with Best Friends Trio (BestFriendsTrio.com).

Ruthanna and husband Roy reside in Anacortes, WA (summers) and Palm Desert, CA (winters). They both are graduates of the Mountaineer's Basic Climbing Course and are avid mountaineers.

For information about starting a *SongShine* program in your area and becoming a certified *SongShine* instructor, please contact her at 425-210-3612 or summitsinger@earthlink.net

Life is But A Weaving

My life is but a weaving
Between my God and me.
I cannot choose the colors
He weaveth steadily.

Oft' times He weaveth sorrow;
And I in foolish pride
Forget He sees the upper
And I the underside.

Not 'til the loom is silent
And the shuttles cease to fly
Will God unroll the canvas
And reveal the reason why.

The dark threads are as needful
In the weaver's skillful hand
As the threads of gold and silver
In the pattern He has planned

He knows, He loves, He cares;
Nothing this truth can dim.
He gives the very best to those
Who leave the choice to Him.

Author Unknown

My Own Thoughts

Loose Threads
Difficult Situations

Each one of us has times in life that cause them to ask:

Why Me?   *Why This?*   *Why Now?*

Can you think of a time when a difficult situation actually turned out to be a blessing in disguise?

_____

_____

_____

_____

_____

_____

_____

_____

_____

_____

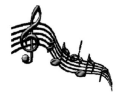